These Fascinating Facts About Drugs that Changed the World?

ASPIRIN, known only since the last half of the 19th century, is derived from the bark of the willow tree. Scientists were looking for a fever-reducing drug to replace quinine, and the search led to the isolation of *acetylsalicylic acid*—aspirin—in 1899.

DIGITALIS, the first miracle drug of modern times, was derived from the common English garden flower foxglove, and discovered over 200 years ago in an herbal potion concocted by an old Shropshire folk healer to treat dropsy (congestive heart failure). But another century and a half would pass before its true value in the treatment of heart disease would be established.

CAFFEINE can be a very important drug for the treatment of premature infants, in whom it reduces the number of apneic (nonbreathing) spells. As the most widely used drug in Western society, caffeine is an effective stimulant, and far safer than amphetamines.

CYCLOSPORINE, the miracle drug that has made organ transplants practical, was discovered by a Swiss microbiologist in 1969, in fungus from a soil sample. First tested on humans in the late 1970s, cyclosporine was the first-ever *selective* immunosuppressant, inhibiting the cells responsible for rejection, while leaving the rest of the immune system relatively intact.

WONDER DRUGS

MARK S. GOLD, M.D.

WITH MICHAEL BOYETTE

PUBLISHED BY POCKET BOOKS NEW YORK

Another *Original* publication of POCKET BOOKS

POCKET BOOKS, a division of Simon & Schuster, Inc.
1230 Avenue of the Americas, New York, N.Y. 10020

Produced by Bookmark Books, Inc.,
Lawrence Chilnick & Bert Stern
Copyright © 1987 by Bookmark Books, Inc.
Cover photograph copyright © 1987 by Al Pisano

ISBN: 0-671-52344-9

First Pocket Books trade paperback printing April, 1987

10 9 8 7 6 5 4 3 2 1

POCKET and colophon are registered trademarks
of Simon & Schuster, Inc.

Printed in the U.S.A.

To Meyer M. Gold

Acknowledgments

There are many people we have to thank for the important contributions they made to this book. First, of course, are the thousands of researchers, physicians, patients, and others who have played a role in the breakthroughs described in this book. Special thanks to my mentors, including: at the University of Florida College of Medicine, Waldo R. Fisher, M.D., Ph.D., Hugh M. Hill, M.D., Steven F. Zornetzer, Ph.D.; at the Yale University School of Medicine, George Aghajanian, M.D., D. Eugene Redmond, Jr., M.D., and George Heninger, M.D.

On a more personal level, we'd like to thank:

Larry Chilnick and Bert Stern, of Bookmark Books, who conceived and developed this project.

We especially thank Randi, Joshua, and Sarah Boyette, whose love, patience, and support helped their father immeasurably.

Our editor, Sydny Weinberg Miner, who has been tireless in her support for this book.

Dan Montopoli, whose research is scattered throughout these pages.

Also, thanks to Ned Leavitt of the William Morris Agency, Barbara Capone, A. Carter Pottash, M.D., and other members of the Fair Oaks staff.

Contents

Foreword

by Mark S. Gold, M.D.

Drugs have come in for a lot of bad publicity in recent years. They don't work, say critics; the drugs are unhealthy or even hazardous. Antipsychotic drugs such as chlorpromazine (Thorazine®) are nothing more than a chemical straitjacket, and oral contraceptives simply a means of exploiting women. Meanwhile, the true path to salvation lies not in drugs, but in carrot juice or a macrobiotic diet, or weight training or yoga.

Is the criticism justified? To a large extent, the answer is no. In fact, much of it is dangerous and irresponsible. Consider, for example, a 1982 network news story on the DPT vaccine, as described in this report from *Medical World News:*

Did DPT Vaccine Get Smeared on National Television?

In January 1981, a man phoned an investigative reporter from Washington's NBC-owned WRC-TV. "I've got a story for you," he said, and proceeded to tell her what happened to his son after a whooping cough vaccination. The result, more than a year later, was "DPT: Vaccine Roulette," an hour-long documentary "exposing" the vaccine's risks, complete with footage of writhing, brain-damaged children.

"DPT: Vaccine Roulette" accomplished its task. It focused national attention on the price a few are paying for a highly effective vaccine that protects most without any problems—a vaccine all believe should be safer. But the program, too, may have exacted a price in suffering. "This program—though it contained some gross misrepresentations—has certainly built a fire under efforts to improve the pertussis vaccine and under the medical profession to more accurately inform patients about its adverse effects," says

11

Dr. M. Harry Jennison, executive director of the American Academy of Pediatrics. "But you can't imagine the sobbing anxiety it's created among young mothers and the tragedy that may occur if immunization is curtailed."

The documentary stated that perhaps one in 700 vaccinated children risks serious reactions from the pertussis part of the vaccine, and many of those reactions may be causing undetected brain damage over and above the obvious neurologic havoc from at least one in 100,000 shots. The report took doctors and the government to task for doing next to nothing about all this, while mandating every child have the shots. It implied some old-boy cover-up of past indiscretions by pediatricians, the CDC, and the FDA.

The next morning, a snippet of the documentary appeared nationwide on NBC's *Today* show. That excerpt sent thousands of American parents to their doctors. The familiar old booster shots suddenly and powerfully had become poison.

Was this journalism at its best, uncovering a clear hazard to the children of America, revealing a gross abuse of trust by pediatricians and the two federal agencies most concerned with protecting the public from epidemics? Or was this just another case of lay reporters, trying hard but failing in their efforts to fathom the depths of epidemiology and the inevitable bad reactions when millions of people are given anything?

"We consider the program to have been distorted, verging on the irresponsible," charged CDC director William H. Foege.

"Attempts are being made to provoke a major controversy where one does not exist."

Pediatrician Edward A. Mortimer Jr., chairman of epidemiology and community health at Cleveland's Case Western Reserve University, was the AAP's spokesman on the documentary, and he came off wearing a black hat. When asked by Lea Thompson, who was the producer-reporter for the show, how a vaccine destined for millions of children could be okayed by merely a three-to-two vote, which an FDA panel—on which Dr. Mortimer sat—did for a DPT vaccine in 1973, the exchange went like this:

Dr. Mortimer: [It was approved] because there was circumstantial evidence that it worked.

Thompson: But a three-to-two vote?

Dr. Mortimer: That's a far greater majority than we elect presidents on.

It smacked of a smart-alecky answer to a serious question, and it didn't look good, admits Dr. Mortimer. Journalists have the obligation to ensure they give a fair report of an interview—conveying both what the person being interviewed wanted to say and what he may have revealed unintentionally. Did Thompson fulfill her obligation?

"Unfair!" cries Dr. Mortimer. Four times, he explained carefully the technical reasons for the three-to-two vote in 1973. Finally, asked a fifth time, he acted flippant in exasperation. That's what got on the air. But Thompson says his previous replies were equally unresponsive.

The show was a "disaster," says Dr. Mortimer. He contends it virtually ignored the hazards of the disease itself (particularly the segment on *Today*) as well as a unanimous consensus of risk-benefit analyses in favor of using the vaccine. It implied unfairly, he contends, that doctors and the government aren't concerned about improving DPT when, in fact, the FDA's Bureau of Biologics has been trying (MWN, April 12, p. 22). Worse, says Dr. Mortimer, the facts were slippery.

For example, he says, the discussion kept sliding from a rate of reaction from the pertussis vaccine (one in 700) to mentions of brain damage from the vaccine (one in 100,000) so that it often seemed the rate of brain damage was far greater than it was. It didn't mention the estimated rate of brain damage from pertussis itself (one in 8,000, according to extrapolations from Swedish and British studies). Thompson says she was unable to obtain that statistic despite many attempts.

Moreover, the only recent U.S. study on reactions to the vaccine, done by Drs. Christopher L. Cody and Larry J. Baraff at UCLA in 1978, and reported in last November's *Pediatrics,* was quoted frequently for its finding of a reaction rate of one in 700. But the program never stated flatly brain damage wasn't found in any of the children. Instead, Thompson suggested some of the reactions can cause brain damage, and said there's been no follow-up to find out whether they did. But, says Dr. Baraff, 12 of the 18 children with reactions within 48 hours were found and reported normal by their parents a year later—though no formal follow-up was done.

Most damning, says Dr. Mortimer, the program omitted the study's conclusion: "Benefits of pertussis immunization far outweigh the risks."

Instead it quoted as an expert Chicago pediatrician and "column doc" Robert S. Mendelsohn as calling DPT "a much greater threat than the whooping cough itself." But the program didn't mention that Dr. Mendelsohn objects to giving children any vaccine—including polio, diphtheria, and tetanus—says Dr. Mortimer. The program identified Dr. Mendelsohn as a one-time pediatrics chief at the University of Illinois, but he wasn't. He was an associate professor for two years until 1971, and, until 1979, an associate professor of preventive medicine.

As to the show in general, says Dr. Mortimer, any benefit it might have in getting the Bureau of Biologics more money to pursue a safer DPT vaccine will be far outweighed by the deaths from pertussis among children whose parents are frightened off the vaccine by unbacked innuendo.

But clearly Thompson hit some raw nerves. Though it was hardly news to pediatricians the vaccine is not as safe as they would like, most of their patients aren't aware of the benefit-risk story.

"It's a terrible problem about how much to tell them," admits Dr. Mortimer. Thompson says only a third of the shots are given by pediatricians, and other physicians may not be so aware of the contraindications after the first shot for the rest.

Thompson says that she was very careful "not to take a point of view as to the risk of the vaccine versus the risk of the disease. That is up to the medical community. Our objective in doing the story was to put forth enough information in order that parents and doctors could have a dialogue on the vaccine."

In fact, "DPT: Vaccine Roulette" made a powerful case for risking the disease rather than having immunization—an assessment hard to avoid from a transcript.

A mother who only sees the show once has no chance to read a transcript carefully, but she remembers the brain-damaged children and their distraught parents. For her, there can be only one conclusion from the documentary—panic.

It illustrates the difficulties of TV journalism and its ephemeral nature. All that can be taken away is a percep-

14

tion: they wouldn't be doing this show unless that stuff is dangerous. The "exposé" revealed the tragedy of brain damage from the vaccine, but it didn't show funerals of children in Britain who have died during a pertussis outbreak since a similar scare discouraged DPT shots there five years ago.

So it's all the more important for TV journalists, whose impact is so powerful, to report matters of public health as even-handedly as possible. "DPT: Vaccine Roulette," for all its good intentions, seems to have tilted too far to risk over benefit.

—Lois Wingerson and
Mark Bloom

The type of sensationalism and inaccuracy described in this report can kill people, by scaring them away from needed medical care. Patients assaulted with misinformation may well come to believe that their doctors are at best ignorant or at worst involved in some great conspiracy with the drug companies to maximize profits at the expense of their patients' health. They may turn to "alternative" treatments that are ineffective or dangerous. They may needlessly suffer or die as a result.

I remember being a resident and hearing a patient say that the AMA blocked new treatments simply to keep doctors in business. If so, they never let me in on the secret. I've read of the "clinics" in Tijuana where cancer is treated with carrot juice and coffee enemas, and the outright lies that some proponents of these "alternative treatments" offer in their defense. One—a physician—recently told a meeting of the "Cancer Control Society" that "the 'proven cures' of the American Cancer Society do not exist"—surprising news, no doubt, to the millions of people in this country who have survived cancer with the help of modern medicine. Another speaker at the same conference claimed that "over three decades the complex of organized medicine, pharmaceutical companies, and government agencies are still using and researching the same fruitless methods for trying to cure cancer." Perhaps he overlooked the exciting new research now being conducted with monoclonal antibodies—substances that didn't even exist a few years ago.

Unfortunately, the list of examples could go on and on, but I think the point is clear. One of the goals of this book is to present a balanced and realistic point of view, and so help consumers make truly informed decisions about their medical care. Its intent is not to suggest that modern medicine has all the answers; in fact, you will find some accounts of spectacular failures—seeming wonder drugs that, for one reason or another, didn't live up to their early promise. Rather, the purpose of *Wonder Drugs* is to help you tell the difference between a real and alleged wonder drug, and also to tell you something about where modern drugs come from, how they work, and how they can improve our lives.

1

What Wonder Drugs Mean to Doctors— and to You

The past fifty years—a mere eyeblink in the history of man—have encompassed a profound revolution in our age-old battle against death and disease. As revolutions go, it's been a rather quiet one, especially considering the stakes involved. There have been no ticker tape parades, and only occasional reports in the daily paper. Only a handful of its heroes are known outside their narrow specialties. Few, if any, kids daydream about joining their ranks.

And yet the pharmaceutical revolution that began with the discovery of penicillin has saved millions of lives and promises to save millions more. In addition, it's changed our view of health and disease, and of doctors and the healing arts. The word "medicine" has two meanings—on the one hand, the work that physicians do, and on the other, the drugs that they dispense. Today more than ever, those two meanings are merging into one.

What Wonder Drugs Mean to Doctors

How, specifically, has the development of these drugs affected physicians? The list could be almost endless, but here are some reflections on the changes they've brought about for my colleagues and me.

First, *wonder drugs change the way doctors treat illness.*
They often offer treatment where *none* was available before;
just as important, they provide alternatives to treatments that
may be painful, disfiguring, or even life-threatening. Before the
advent of effective antiulcer medications, the treatment of
choice for ulcers was surgery—actually cutting out the part of
the stomach that was diseased. Before the discovery of immunosuppressive drugs, the only treatment for kidney failure was
dialysis. In addition, wonder drugs represent an improvement
over earlier drug treatments that had too many side effects or
too few responders. In earlier times, some "cures" were worse
than the disease—the use of cocaine suppositories for hemorrhoids, for instance, or arsenic for syphilis.

Even when they don't cure a disease, wonder drugs can
often restore a diseased organ to marginal or even good function and so forestall or postpone more dangerous types of
therapy. Digitalis, for instance, doesn't cure heart failure the
way a heart transplant can, but can make the diseased heart
work well enough that a heart transplant isn't needed.

Wonder drugs have made the role of the individual physi-
cian less important. Increasingly, doctors are *vehicles,* whose
role is simply to get the right drug to the right patient in time for
it to do some good. Many physicians will take issue with this
view, but to my mind it's a positive development. Certainly
wonder drugs don't detract from the skill of the most gifted
doctors at the most up-to-date medical centers; wonder drugs
simply make it possible for other doctors to obtain equally
spectacular results.

Wonder drugs change the way doctors diagnose illness. In
the old days, diagnosis wasn't as important as it is now. If you
diagnosed stomach cancer and your patient really had liver
cancer, it didn't make much difference. In either event there
was nothing you could do, and the outcome was likely to be the
same. In fact, sometimes doctors tended to favor one diagnosis
over another simply because certain conditions were hopeless.
Before the advent of lithium therapy, for example, psychiatrists
avoided the diagnosis of manic-depressive illness in favor of
schizophrenia, since the former was a virtual death sentence.
As long as manic-depressive disorders were untreatable, arguably little harm was done; today, however, it's become essential
for psychiatrists to clearly differentiate between these two disorders.

Wonder drugs help doctors understand why certain dis- ses occur. Very often in pharmacology, drugs are found to be ective before anyone can explain why. As further research ktracks in an attempt to explain these agents' effectiveness, often gain important insights into the workings of the body. r example, the discovery of endorphins—substances within e brain that seem to regulate pleasure and pain—resulted m investigations of how narcotics work.

Wonder drugs can change—even create—entire medical iplines. Witness the changes in the field of psychiatry, for ple. Not so many years ago, psychiatry was almost ex- ely concerned with such mysterious entities as the id and perego, and was considered by many to be a sort of ild of medicine. Today it's up to its ego in biochemistry ares a great deal of common ground with such main- specialties as internal medicine and neurology. In large change is due to a single drug: chlorpromazine (Thor- By demonstrating that psychiatric symptoms could be ed by chemical means, this drug demonstrated that s of the mind are in fact caused by *physical* disorders the brain. The field of oncology—the treatment of can- s another example. It's a relatively new specialty in medi- cine, and to a large extent it owes its existence to the various anticancer drugs that have been developed in this century.

Finally, *wonder drugs make the practice of medicine more enjoyable.* There's nothing a physician hates more than being unable to help a sick or dying patient. By the same token, there's nothing that makes us feel as good as restoring some- one's well-being. In my own practice, I've seen former nar- cotics addicts—sick, malnourished, unable to hold a conversation, much less a job—put their lives back together with the help of a drug called naltrexone. My colleagues in cardiology see heart-attack patients survive and become healthy thanks to beta-blockers and other heart medications: grandmothers who go on to become great-grandmothers; young men who return to their families, jobs, and lives; suc- cessful men and women who continue to contribute to our world and savor life perhaps more than ever. Wonder drugs make it possible to treat such formerly untreatable diseases as childhood leukemia, Hodgkin's disease, and multiple myeloma. These are the sorts of successes that make it worth coming to work every morning.

How Wonder Drugs Affect People

There are additional ways, not often considered, in which these drugs affect us all, patients and physicians alike:

Wonder drugs make medicine more affordable. Not only are drugs usually less dangerous than surgery or other alternatives to treatment, they're also considerably less expensive. Beta-blocker therapy may cost a few hundred dollars a year—a mere fraction of the cost of a single day in a coronary care unit. Cyclosporine, one of the most expensive drugs on the market, may cost several thousand dollars a year for the typical renal-transplant patient—a lot of money, perhaps, but still less expensive than dialysis. In the final analysis, wonder drugs may be the most effective means we have of controlling the costs of medical care.

Wonder drugs make it possible to regulate medicine. A hundred years ago there was hardly any regulation of medical care, either by the government or by anyone else. Part of the reason was the laissez-faire philosophy of the nineteenth century, but part was because the medicine of that day was, by and large, a hit-or-miss affair. Wonder drugs have helped make regulation possible because they help make treatment predictable. We know that it usually takes a certain number of days to clear up a staph infection; we know that the typical length of stay in a hospital after a heart attack is no more than two or three weeks. We know how much a drug costs, and we know what the usual dosage is. Thus, it's possible to come up with fairly accurate estimates of the costs of treating various diseases. This predictability, in turn, makes it possible for health insurers to estimate their projected payouts, and so set premiums. It also makes possible such cost-controlling schemes as Medicare's diagnosis-related group (DRG) system, which pays hospitals a predetermined amount of money to treat a patient with a given diagnosis.

Wonder drugs give more people access to the best medicine has to offer. In the medical world, the superstars are usually surgeons—doctors such as William deVries and Christiaan Barnard—for the simple reason that success in surgery depends greatly on the doctor's skill. Wonder drugs, however, work just as well no matter who prescribes them. The doctor's skill is still important, of course, for proper diagnosis and monitoring, but even so, these drugs greatly improve the quality of care for most patients—regardless of who their doctor is.

Wonder drugs make medicine more of a science, and less of an art, for many of the reasons we've already mentioned. They make it easier for doctors to know when new "breakthroughs" truly represent progress over already established treatments. It's possible, for instance, to conduct drug trials that clearly and objectively demonstrate how a new drug compares with other therapy. In this way, they're much easier to evaluate than, say, a new surgical technique that may depend on an individual surgeon's skill, or a counseling program that cannot easily be reproduced in various settings.

Wonder drugs make medical care more available and convenient. They reduce the need for patients and their families to travel long distances for treatment. For many conditions, the best in modern medicine is no further away than the corner drugstore, and when a condition is treatable with drugs, patients in the smallest and most rural communities can receive care as good as any they could get at a big-city hospital. Likewise, the relatively low cost and widespread availability of wonder drugs mean that the best medical care isn't limited to a wealthy minority. Penicillin—which has saved countless lives and is arguably the most important drug ever discovered—costs only a few dollars per prescription and is available anywhere.

Finally, wonder drugs create hope. Many "hopeless" diseases have already been conquered by wonder drugs, and these successes justify our hope of conquering the illnesses that continue to plague us. Indeed, wonder drugs have altered the way we view disease itself. Disease is no longer quite so fearsome as it once was; time and again, it has yielded to our efforts to overcome it. This spiritual victory is not always obvious, but it may well be the most important victory of all.

2

Of Wonders
and Miracles

Imagine a world where half the people born every year never live to see their fortieth birthday, a world where epidemics come in waves, tumbling one upon another so quickly that people aren't even sure of the name of the disease they're dying from. Imagine wounded soldiers by the millions, losing limbs and lives not in the fury of battle, but in crowded and stinking hospitals, dying inch by inch to the onslaught of gangrene and infection. Imagine a culture so obsessed with death that its ideal of beauty is the pale and wasted frame of the tuberculosis patient, and its idea of relaxation a Sunday outing to the cemetery.

Imagine doctors haunted by the screams of their patients, turning pale at the thought of performing an operation, condemning countless patients with the words, "There's nothing I can do." Imagine patients unable to move their swollen bodies, or locked away in dark places for their entire lives.

These are not nightmares, or medieval visions of hell; they are all scenes of everyday life in the not-so-distant past—a past having no penicillin, no anesthesia—not even simple aspirin. It was a world dominated by pain, disease, and premature death, ruled by ignorance and fear.

This book is about wonder drugs and miracle drugs—those substances that have in large part erased such horrors from our lives and even from our consciousness. It's about the brightest stars of modern pharmaceutical science, those drugs that rate an A+ for their effectiveness and safety.

But what, precisely, is a wonder drug? What's a miracle drug? And what's the difference between the two?

Let's start with wonder drug, a term that can't be defined precisely, of course, for everyone has different ideas of what these drugs are and what they're supposed to do. To the research doctor, for example, some new experimental compound that offers a slight but consistent reduction in the death rate among cancer patients might qualify. An up-and-coming executive plagued by severe dandruff might look upon an effective dandruff shampoo as a very different kind of wonder drug. What is the common thread between these two extremes?

A dictionary-style definition probably isn't possible, but here are some rules of thumb we can follow in deciding whether a particular drug is "wondrous":

Rule 1: Wonder drugs work whether you believe in them or not. Once upon a time—not so long ago, actually—there was a doctor with a reputation for being *the* best name in the treatment of manic-depressive illness. His office walls were papered with diplomas, certificates, and awards; his nurses and fellow physicians spoke of him in tones of reverence and awe; his waiting room was full of eager patients; his files were bulging with success stories. He could, it seemed, work wonders where others had failed. More than anything else, his secret of success was that his patients *believed* in him.

In the city where he practiced, he'd virtually cornered the market on manic-depressive illness—until doctors learned to treat the disorder with lithium. Suddenly, it didn't matter whether you believed in your treatment or your doctor; a round of lithium therapy and your spirits began to take a turn for the better. The result? The "manic-depressive illness specialist" began treating schizophrenia.

It's undeniably true that good health and a good attitude have a lot to do with each other. But even so, wonder drugs don't depend upon a doctor's charisma or persuasiveness, nor on the patient's desire to get better. They work when the physician has a lousy bedside manner, and they work when he's off vacationing in Florida. They work whether you go to a run-down clinic or a fancy private office. They work even if you don't want them to work—as is the case with naltrexone, which keeps addicts from getting high no matter how much heroin they shoot up. Wonder drugs cure cancer even when the patient and his family think the doctor's simply lying in an attempt to put their minds at ease. They make you feel better even if your therapist tells you that you haven't gotten in touch with your feelings, or your chiropractor tells you your spine's out of alignment.

This rule suggests another, related one:

Rule 2: Wonder drugs have been proven effective by published, verifiable scientific studies. Before a new drug—any new drug—is approved by the Food and Drug Administration (FDA) for use in the United States, its manufacturer must submit the results of extensive scientific studies to demonstrate its safety and effectiveness. To be sure, this process isn't foolproof. Some drugs turn out to have adverse side effects, for instance, which occur so rarely that they're overlooked in the preliminary studies, and sometimes the studies are tainted by the manufacturer's eagerness to have the drug approved. But even with these flaws, this process means you can be pretty sure that a drug approved by the FDA is effective. By contrast, you'll usually find that unsupported testimonials and attacks on mainstream medicine are the sole basis for the "wonder drug" status of such substances as laetrile.

The promoters of laetrile, for example, would have you believe that there's some sinister conspiracy between doctors and the big drug companies to keep this "wonder drug" out of the hands of dying patients. But the argument just doesn't ring true. Every doctor we've ever met would jump at the chance to prescribe a drug that offered any value, no matter how slight, to a terminal cancer patient and there's probably not a single pharmaceutical company executive who hasn't dreamed of discovering and marketing a new cure for cancer—no matter where it comes from.

But, say some critics, drug companies are only interested in drugs that can be patented, since profits are so much higher when competition is eliminated. That, these critics say, is the real reason that drug companies won't sell laetrile.

Well, it's true that a drug company would *prefer* to have a patent on some amazing new drug—who wouldn't?—but it doesn't follow that they're *only* interested in such agents. You can make aspirin in any high school chemistry lab, and the patent on it expired long ago, but does that mean drug companies aren't interested in selling it? A stroll through any drug store suggests otherwise.

None of this is to say, however, that only FDA-approved drugs work. There are many promising but unproven compounds that are, at this very moment, undergoing extensive testing and investigation; we'll even be examining a number of these in the chapters to come. But a quick look at any pharmaceutical text from twenty years ago will reveal that promise is one thing and proof is another. Realistically speaking, many of the avenues now being pursued by researchers will turn out to be blind alleys, and for that reason we've been careful to distinguish in this book between *proven* wonder drugs and *possible* wonder drugs.

Rule 3: Wonder drugs offer real benefits, not trivial or illusory ones. That's a tough call sometimes and depends on a number of factors. For one thing, it varies from person to person: A particularly well-adjusted teenager, for instance, might view her acne as a bothersome but not too important side effect of adolescence, while many others experience a devastation whose emotional scars are likely to be as deep and as ugly as their physical ones. In such cases, a drug like Accutane® is a wonder drug because it promises a significant improvement in the quality of people's lives.

Rule 4: Wonder drugs are those whose benefits clearly outweigh their drawbacks. At times—with some anticancer drugs, for instance—a drug's side effects or other drawbacks can be severe, but its benefits are so great that it's worth it. Sometimes a drug is a wonder drug because it offers the benefits of an earlier wonder drug *without* its problems—as we'll see with calcium-channel blockers, for instance. Sometimes the benefit offered by a wonder drug is not earth-shattering (let's face it, nobody ever died of dandruff), but the drug is so inexpensive and safe that we're all still better off for having it around.

Rule 5: Wonder drugs are here for the long haul. They are not pharmaceutical fads or fashions, to be tossed out like yesterday's newspaper. They're drugs that will be around for the next twenty, thirty, or even a hundred years—unless they're supplanted by new, improved versions or, like the smallpox vaccine, are so successful that they put themselves out of a job.

These characteristics pretty well sum up wonder drugs, but we still haven't talked about wonder drugs versus miracle drugs. Although to most people the terms are interchangeable, for our purposes there is a distinction. Miracle drugs possess all the qualities of wonder drugs, but they also have something extra. They change the way we look at disease; their discovery opens up whole new areas of medicine.

Miracle drugs are like vision restored to a blind man; they are to medicine what Bach was to music or what Einstein was to physics. They are the pharmaceutical equivalent of the flash of inspiration or stroke of genius, the sunlight at the break of day. They transform the world.

Think back to the examples at the beginning of this chapter. Penicillin and sulfa drugs didn't simply provide a new way to treat infections; they represented the first time doctors could treat infections at all. Ether didn't just make it easier to perform operations; it changed, fundamentally and forever, the role that surgery was to play in medicine.

Miracle drugs may actually provide a clue as to why an illness occurs and start us on the way to a deeper understanding of the disease process. Almost overnight, they can make standard therapies obsolete, emptying tuberculosis sanatoriums and leper colonies. Once they arrive, it seems they've been here forever, and we can barely remember the way things used to be.

3

Miracles from Mold: Antibiotics

If you were to ask a group of doctors to name the single most significant drug in the history of medicine, chances are good that nearly all of them would give you the same answer: penicillin.

Why? In part because of the millions of lives it's saved and the many diseases it's tamed. In part because it created a whole new class of drugs, and pointed the way toward development of other drugs as diverse as streptomycin and cyclosporine. But even more important is the fact that its discovery marked a profound change in the role that drugs play in the treatment of disease. Penicillin represented the first major discovery of a drug that *cured* disease.

Consider for a moment what that means. As late as 1943, doctors had no significant drugs that cured disease. They had vaccines that could *prevent* disease, and they had other drugs—digitalis, for instance—that could relieve some of the *symptoms* of disease. They had skillful surgical techniques that could, to a certain extent, repair the damage done by disease. They even had drugs—sulfa drugs—that could slow the spread of bacterial infection and thus give the body's immune system a fighting chance to recover. But they had no drug that could, in and of itself, *conquer* disease.

In those days, doctors could handle such things as broken bones and births nearly as well as their counterparts today. But for many diseases they could do little more than keep patients as comfortable as possible while waiting for them to die or get better on their own.

And then, suddenly, from Alexander Fleming's laboratory dish emerged a substance he wasn't even looking for, one that within a few years would conquer an amazing array of diseases, from blood poisoning to postsurgical infection.

Bacteria: The Invisible Killers

These diseases and the others cured by penicillin have one thing in common: they occur when the body is invaded by millions of harmful bacteria. Not all diseases are caused by bacteria, of course, but such deadly ones as blood poisoning, cholera, and tuberculosis are. These are the diseases against which the antibiotics—penicillin, erythromycin, and tetracycline, to name a few—are effective.

To understand why, we must start with some definitions from the world of microbiology. *Microbes* are the tiny organisms you probably remember viewing through the microscope in biology class. *Cultures* are colonies of microbes that are grown in the laboratory—typically in small glass dishes known as *Petri dishes*—to study the organisms' properties. The organisms may be any of various types, such as *fungi* (singular, fungus), which are microscopic cousins of the mushrooms; *amoebae* (singular, amoeba)—the oozy, octopuslike cells that many people think of when we speak of microscopic life; and *bacteria,* among others.

There are countless species of bacteria (if it's only one, it's called a bacterium), but they all share certain features. The most important for our purposes is their tough "skin" or *cell wall;* it encloses the cell and protects it from the outside environment. Because of this cell wall, bacteria have well-defined shapes, and scientists classify them according to their shape: spherical ones are termed *cocci* (singular, coccus); rod-shaped ones are called *bacilli* (singular, bacillus); and twisted ones are known as *spirilla* (singular, spirillum).

The microscopic world also includes *viruses*—primitive structures that fall in the gray area between living and nonliving objects. Like all living organisms, they are able to reproduce themselves, but they can only do so with the assistance of another organism, which is often destroyed in the process. Viruses are much smaller than bacteria—so tiny, in fact, that they can't be seen under an ordinary microscope. *Pathogens* are microbes or viruses that cause disease; germs, in layman's terms.

Now, armed with these definitions, let's take a closer look at bacteria. Not all of them are pathogens; in fact, the vast majority are harmless or even beneficial to humans. For instance, at this very moment there are several million bacteria making their home in your stomach and intestines. They started to move in a few hours after you were born, and they (actually, their descendants) have been there ever since.

Most of these bacteria are of an amiable sort known as *Escherichia coli*—or *E. coli* for short. They live off bits of food that your stomach and intestines can't absorb, and ordinarily they don't cause any harm. In fact, they're decidedly friendly; they fight off unfamiliar and unwanted microbes that show up in their neighborhood from time to time.

Bacteria are everywhere—in the air, in the soil, in our food and water, but most, fortunately, are as harmless as *E. coli* usually is. Only a relative handful of species cause diseases.

And contrary to what you might think, even they aren't all that harmful except in relatively rare instances. After all, we're exposed every day to the bacteria that cause infection, pneumonia, blood poisoning, even cholera and tuberculosis, and most of the time we don't fall prey to them.

The reason is that Mother Nature has given us some very effective defenses against these microscopic bad guys. The skin forms a first line of defense, preventing airborne bacteria from entering the body. The few that do slip through—say, through a cut—are faced with an even more formidable threat: the immune system, a kind of police force that watches for foreign invaders. Intruders trigger a chemical alarm that calls up white blood cells (they're really transparent, but they're called white to distinguish them from oxygen-transporting red blood cells), which promptly dispose of the threat by eating the unwelcome guests.

Almost always, the immune system successfully protects us from disease. Sometimes, if the invasion is extensive, some time elapses before the invaders are repelled. In the meantime, we feel sick—but still we shouldn't be too quick to blame the germ. The fever that almost always accompanies an infection, for instance, is created not by pathogens but by the immune system, and it seems to have something to do with the body's

The "Bubble Boy": A Body at the Mercy of the World

A normally functioning immune system permits us to live in a world full of hostile microbes. Its importance is illustrated by the story of David, a Houston boy who spent his entire life inside a germ-free plastic bubble.

Shortly after he was born, David (his last name has always been withheld by his parents for reasons of privacy) was diagnosed as suffering from *severe combined immune deficiency (SCID)*. Approximately one child in a million is born with this disease, which until very recently was always fatal. SCID children are born without an immune system, leaving their bodies prey to any disease that they encounter.

David's doctors knew that they had no cure for his disease. But in the hopes that a cure might become available, they decided to buy time by placing the child in isolation—first in a special incubator, and later in an *isolation room*. These superclean rooms are used for patients who are at high risk for infection—for example, burn patients, whose damaged skin permits pathogens to enter the body easily. Isolation rooms have special air conditioning systems with air filters that can trap even microscopic organisms. The rooms are pressurized so that if a door is opened, air flows out of the room rather than into it. For isolation patients, everything brought into the room—instruments, bed linens, even dinner dishes—must first be sterilized. Doctors, nurses, and visitors who enter the room must wear surgical gowns and masks, and must "scrub up" as if they're about to enter an operating room.

After he spent several months in this sterile prison, David's plight came to the attention of NASA officials at the nearby Houston Space Center. During the Apollo project, NASA had developed a great deal of expertise in isolation techniques, for a very unusual reason: an extremely remote but potentially devastating possibility that the astronauts might pick up an extraterrestrial pathogen during their trips to the moon and back. Nobody really thought that such bugs existed, but to be on the safe side, NASA scientists had developed an elaborate quarantine system for returning astronauts to ensure that any alien diseases would not spread to the population at large.

In David's case the problem was reversed—it was he who needed protection from the outside world—but the techniques were similar. NASA built David a special plastic bubble in the hospital, and when he outgrew that one, they built him a larger one for home.

Thus began what amounted to a life sentence for little David. As he grew up in the bubble, he looked and acted like any normal child. But his existence was far from normal: He never touched another person except through the plastic barrier of his bubble, and everything he came into contact with required sterilization—his clothes and toys, his meals, even the closed-circuit television by which he participated in his elementary school classes. He could leave his tiny world only by donning a spacesuit-like outfit that, like his bubble, shielded him from the world. As it confined his life, the bubble shaped his dreams—his ambition, he said, was to someday walk through wet grass in his bare feet.

When David was twelve, his doctors presented his parents with a choice: Take a chance on a new therapy or let David continue to live in the bubble. The therapy involved the transplant of bone marrow from a donor.

After talking it over with David, his parents agreed to try the risky technique. At last David entered the world that had been, for him, as alien and hostile as the surface of the moon. He received the bone-marrow transplant, but it was no use; within days of leaving the shelter of his bubble, David was dead. Doctors found massive tumors throughout his body, caused, they believed, by invading viruses.

At a news conference shortly after David's death, his doctor said that despite David's death, bone-marrow transplants were the only real hope for children with SCID. But now that the treatment was available, he said, such children would be treated as soon as the disease was diagnosed. There would be no more "bubble children."

fight against an infection. Doctors aren't sure just what role fever plays; one thought is that it is an attempt to make the body a less pleasant place for temperature-sensitive pathogens.

In the ordinary course of events, the white blood cells eventually gain the upper hand, the crisis passes, and life goes on as before. But not always. At times, the bacteria may breach the body's normal defenses—say, through an open wound—and enter in overwhelming numbers. Or, if the body is in a weakened state, the immune system may be impaired and easily overcome.

Often, these two factors go hand in hand—a surgical incision may provide a point of entry for bacteria, while the underlying condition that made the operation necessary has diminished the body's defenses. Or a bullet may introduce bacteria, while at the same time causing extensive blood loss that can undermine the body's ability to fight off the infection.

Problems can also arise if the immune system itself is out of kilter. As we'll see in Chapter 9, infection is a major concern in organ transplants, because doctors must "turn off" the immune system, which otherwise would view the new organ as a "foreigner" and destroy it. Certain types of diseases, such as acquired immune deficiency syndrome (AIDS) and severe combined immune deficiency (SCID) also result in a shutdown of the immune system. When, for whatever reason, the immune system isn't working, the body is vulnerable to invasion by just about any organism that happens to come along. Under such circumstances, the normally harmless *E. coli,* for instance, can travel beyond its habitat in the intestines and cause meningitis or urinary tract infections.

It is in circumstances such as these that antibiotics have come to play such an important role. In the past, an infection that overwhelmed the body's natural defenses resulted in almost certain death; now, doctors have an extensive arsenal that, in the vast majority of cases, can tip the scales back toward life.

Penicillin: The Scourge of Bacteria

Alexander Fleming's discovery of penicillin is one of the legends of the modern age—a folk tale, almost, about the value of close observation and overlooked miracles. Countless schoolchildren learn the familiar story—how during the summer of 1929, Fleming—an unknown microbiologist at St. Mary's Hospital in London—undertook a series of experiments using cultures of the deadly staphylococcus bacteria; how, during the cool, damp evenings of that summer, spores of a common mold floated into the laboratory and landed in the bacteria cultures, "ruining" the experiment; how Fleming, about to discard the cultures, happened to notice that the bacteria nearest the mold had mysteriously died, and so, by his quick thinking and keen eye, literally saved this miracle of modern science from the drain of his laboratory sink.

Upon hearing the story, you're left with the impression that this happy accident instantaneously transformed the world from a place of ignorance to one of hope. But what's usually left out of this tale is the ending. Did Fleming, upon discovering penicillin, run out into the streets of London, lab coat flapping in the breeze, and announce to passersby that he had saved the world? No; much work would remain to be done before penicillin's potential was fully realized.

In fact, at first Fleming didn't even know what he was working with; when he showed a sample of the mold to a fungus expert, he was told it was a red brush fungus, *Penicillium rubrum*. Only years later would scientists determine that the mold was actually a cousin of the red brush fungus, *Penicillium notatum*.

More important was the fact that the penicillin that Fleming had discovered was very impure, unstable, and difficult to collect. Because of these drawbacks—and, perhaps, because Fleming was a bacteriologist and not a physician, he first used the miracle mold not to cure infection but for the much more mundane task of isolating bacteria in the laboratory. And although this new technique was an important advance in his field, it really didn't do much for patients. Doctors at St. Mary's were intrigued by Fleming's discovery, but neither they nor Fleming himself were willing to use the impure broth in patients. Occasionally, doctors at the hospital applied it to infected wounds, but the effects were too weak and unpredictable to be of much practical use.

All of this was so discouraging that, after eight months, the bacteriologist decided to stop studying his new discovery and simply write a paper summarizing his findings. The report, published in a British scientific journal, carried a long and unpromising title: "On the Anti-bacterial Action of Cultures of a Penicillium, with Special Reference to Their Use in the Isolation of B. Influenza." The most he was willing to say about penicillin was this: "It is suggested that it may be an efficient antiseptic for application to, or injection into, areas infected with penicillin-sensitive microbes."

But even that modest statement was met with skepticism. A famous scientist of the day had this to say about the future of penicillin:

> The penicillium molds are pleasant enough and we are content to use them to bring our Camembert and Roquefort cheeses into a pleasant condition of ripeness, and in that respect I would not like to miss them. But beyond that, and especially with a view to therapy in medicine, these molds are completely useless.

More than eight years would pass before this obituary for penicillin was proved wrong. A two-year series of experiments at the University of London resulted in another dead end, as researchers despaired of finding a way to isolate pure penicillin. For years, the mold lay dormant in Fleming's laboratory, until a group of scientists at Oxford University began to study it anew. This time they succeeded in isolating pure penicillin, and at last doctors had a substance that they could put to the test.

And none too soon, for it was 1939 and the Second World War was beginning. As the armies of Europe met on the battlefield, scientists throughout the world waged their own war against mankind's oldest and most potent enemies: the microbes that caused gangrene, pneumonia, and other infectious diseases. At Oxford, work proceeded quickly but with caution—first, a series of animal experiments that showed penicillin to be nontoxic, and then a test of its effectiveness. Researchers infected eight rats with a virulent strain of bacteria, and then treated half of them with penicillin. The four that went untreated were dead within a day; the four that received penicillin were alive. Further animal studies showed penicillin to be equally effective against many other species of bacteria.

At last the stage was set for studies in man. But the scientists ran into another snag: the glass Petri dishes they'd been using to prepare penicillin were too small to produce the quantities necessary for human experiments. And with a war on, they were unable to obtain larger ones. They tried metal dishes, but soon learned that the metal destroyed the penicillin. Finally, with all the resourcefulness of career quartermasters, they found, practically in their own backyard, plentiful and perfectly suited substitutes: oddly shaped pans large enough for their experiments and coated with protective enamel. Thus did penicillin, the savior of mankind, emerge from years of oblivion, born again in the depths of a hospital bedpan.

Two and a half years would pass until, in August, 1943, the experiments were completed and penicillin became widely available. Its effects on the injured soldiers were immediate and profound. For soldiers suffering stomach wounds, for instance, the survival rate was about 70 percent during World War II. In the Korean War, for which penicillin and other antibiotics were widely available, the rate rose to almost 100 percent.

Penicillin and the Romans

Were the antibiotic properties of the penicillium molds known to the Romans nearly two thousand years before Fleming's famous discovery? That possibility is raised by a small stone rod found by archaeologists during the excavation of a Roman military hospital in Germany. Carved in mirror-image fashion on the rod was a curious inscription:

C. XANTHI PENICILLE AD IMPetum

C. XANTHI DIAMISUS AD ASPeritudinem

Archaeologists have found hundreds of such rods in other excavations, and they believe the Romans used them to label medicinal ointments. The rods, they surmise, were pressed into the soft, pastelike ointments, where they left behind an impression describing the medicine and its uses. The rods that have been found all follow the same format, and so archaeologists studying this particular one were able to decipher the meaning of the inscription.

"C. XANTHI" is the name of the physician who prepared the ointment—sort of an ancient trademark. The word "PENICILLE" appears in the position typically reserved for ingredients. The inscription's second line refers to *vitriol diamisus ad asperitudinem*, a preparation used for eye inflammations.

Can we deduce from this that the Romans possessed an antibiotic eye ointment containing penicillin? The idea is not as far-fetched as it sounds. To the ancient Romans, "penicille" had two meanings—"small brush" and "mold" (because growths of mold often resemble the bristles of a brush). In addition, the stone from which the stamp was carved apparently came from Bavaria, whose inhabitants possessed remarkable insights into the causes and cures of disease. For example, the ancient Bavarians spoke of invisible "worms" as the cause of infection, and they were well acquainted with molds and their value in the treatment of disease. In fact, the physician himself may well have been a native of the area—*Xanthus* means "blond" and was a term that Romans often used to refer to Germans. Thus, it's not impossible that an ancient Bavarian doctor in the service of the Roman army carried with him a folk remedy derived from common molds.

But couldn't the find be a hoax? Not likely; archaeologists discovered the stamp a full thirty years before the world ever heard of Alexander Fleming and the substance he called penicillin.

"Life Hinders Life"

The effectiveness of penicillin demonstrates a profound principle, one that underlies many of the pharmaceutical discoveries of the twentieth century. It was first put forth by Louis Pasteur, who stated it thusly: "Life hinders life."

That may sound like some mystical mantra from the Far East, but it is firmly grounded in the theory of evolution and modern science's understanding of how organisms adapt to their environment. Pasteur, the man who proved that diseases can be caused by bacteria, was talking about microbes, but the principle also holds true in more familiar surroundings.

Experienced gardeners, for instance, know to keep their plants as far as possible from black walnut trees. There are several obvious reasons: trees block sunlight, and their roots draw nutrients out of the soil. But there's another factor that makes black walnuts particularly troublesome: they actually secrete a chemical that stunts the growth of fast-growing competitors. This substance is also present in their leaves, which, when they fall on the ground beneath the tree, kill off any plants that might be growing there.

You can see how this chemical gives the tree a competitive edge in the plant world. In the forest, especially, there are many fast-growing trees and shrubs that, left to themselves, would quickly overtake the stately but slow-growing black walnut. The natural weed-killer that it secretes, however, provides an advantage by choking off potential competitors for water, light, and nutrients. In that way it serves an important evolutionary purpose.

This was precisely the effect noted by Pasteur on the microscopic level. It's a universal law of nature—not only for trees and microbes, but for animals and men as well—that organisms growing near one another tend to develop very specific means of dealing with these competitors. In other words, "life hinders life."

What that means is that if you're looking for a way to control an organism—whether weeds or bacteria—a good place to start is right next door. Pasteur and others who followed him recognized the implications of this principle, and in the century before Fleming's discovery many had looked for a microbe that would prevent the growth of the disease-causing bacteria. In fact, they'd found one—pyocyanase—in 1889 that worked wonderfully in the glass dishes of the laboratory. The problem was that it was just as toxic to man as it was to pathogens.

Fleming, as a bacteriologist who was intimately familiar with Pasteur and his followers, was no doubt aware of the ongoing search for the first "antibiotic"—the name already given to the still-undiscovered substances. And it was doubtless this awareness that made him stop and take a second look at his ruined experiment, and to grasp the significance of what he saw. Thus, it was not simple luck that brought penicillin to the world; it was luck combined with Fleming's keen eye and thorough scientific background.

How Penicillin Works

What is this wondrous chemical that molds produce to fight off competitive bacteria? As drugs go, it's a relatively simple compound, made up of carbon, hydrogen, oxygen, nitrogen, and sulfur atoms. From a pharmacologic point of view, its most significant and useful feature is not that it kills bacteria—many things do that, from alcohol to boiling water—but that it does so within the human body and, for most people, without any ill effects.

Penicillin circulates in the bloodstream, practically inert until it comes upon bacteria. Then it goes to work.

You'll remember that bacteria are surrounded by a tough coating known as a cell wall, whose primary function is to hold the cell together. When the cell is getting ready to divide in two, the cell wall undergoes certain chemical changes, and it is at this point that penicillin mounts its attack. The reproduction of the cell wall involves three carefully orchestrated chemical steps, but just as the process is nearly complete, penicillin sneaks in and chemically pulls the rug out from under the reaction.

The effect on the bacterial cell is immediate and devastating. With its protective "skin" suddenly gone, the cell literally bursts apart, its contents scattered into the surrounding fluid.

There are two things about this mechanism that are of additional clinical significance. First is that it's selective. The body's cells don't have cell walls, which is why the drug doesn't destroy them along with the bacteria. And not all cell walls are

37

the same. Some types of bacteria have cell walls that are immune to the effects of penicillin, which is why it doesn't work against all bacterial infections.

Second, penicillin is only effective against cells that are actively dividing, since it interferes with cell-wall chemistry at that point. That's why doctors tell you to take penicillin even after the symptoms of an infection have cleared up: in all probability living bacteria still remain but are relatively inactive, and the penicillin won't work against them until they begin to divide.

The Problem of Resistance

Pasteur's maxim is a two-way street: organisms that are being "hindered" often respond by "hindering" back. In other words, organisms that are threatened respond with countermeasures. In response to the long teeth and sharp claws of a predator, other species of animals develop swifter legs or longer horns. Such biological battles go back and forth, but the changes are so gradual that they typically don't become apparent for thousands or even millions of years.

Some organisms reproduce so rapidly, however, that this evolutionary process is compressed into a matter of years. Certain types of insects, for example, have already evolved defenses against insecticides, such as DDT, introduced as late as the 1940s while more slowly evolving creatures such as birds and humans are as susceptible as ever to the harmful effects of insecticides.

While insects typically need a few weeks to reproduce, microbes are even more prolific; they can divide in a matter of minutes. Thus, you'd expect to see them evolve defenses against antibiotics that much more quickly—and in fact, many of them do.

Consider what, say, the staphylococcus bacterium—the organism responsible for septic pneumonia and certain other types of infections—is up against in its desperate fight for survival against penicillin. For millions of years, it was able to survive by infecting human beings. There was, of course, the ever-present threat of white blood cells, but even so, the bacteria had managed to do quite well once they became established.

Suddenly, along comes penicillin, the staphylococcal equivalent of the Black Death. This is no minor threat; it's a fight for survival of the entire species. The drug is a formidable opponent since it doesn't simply weaken the bacteria so that the white blood cells can attack, it actually dissolves the cell. When it's finished, there's nothing left but a microscopic puddle of organic chemicals.

And yet, even against such a terrible threat, and without the benefit of the pharmaceutical researchers and laboratories that mankind has at its disposal, the tenacious staphylococci have in a few short decades developed some effective defenses against penicillin.

The fact that they've done so has created some problems for physicians and patients, and it has troubling implications for the future. At the same time, though, it offers perhaps the best corroboration of Darwin's theory of evolution. Here's why:

By and large, staphylococci are all pretty much alike. The reason is their means of reproduction: they simply split in two, and the two resulting cells are, in theory, identical twins. When these twins divide, you end up with four identical organisms; when they divide again, eight, and so on.

If we trace this process backward through time to some mythical Adam/Eve of the staphylococci, you can see that all of the "children" should be absolutely identical to one another. But for a number of reasons, that's not so. Sometimes cells divide imperfectly, and sometimes they undergo changes— mutations—caused by radiation or other environmental factors. These occurrences are relatively rare, but over time they have introduced variations among the staphylococci.

Now suppose that within this great family of staphylococci there's one set of cousins that has the odd ability to withstand penicillin. Perhaps this capability evolved slowly among staphylococci that naturally grew in the vicinity of such molds. Perhaps only a tiny proportion of all staphylococci—say one in a billion—have this special property. In the past, this characteristic had little or no effect on the cell's ability to survive in the human body; it was, for practical purposes, an "invisible" trait.

Suddenly comes the discovery of penicillin—Armageddon for the staphylococci. When the drug is given to an infected patient, all but the few penicillin-resistant staphylococci are killed. The survivors are few in number, but they reproduce rapidly. The result: Within a few years doctors are faced with the problem of treating "new" strains of penicillin-resistant staphylococci.

This is natural selection in action: A change in the environment—that is, the widespread introduction of penicillin—tips the scales in favor of particular bacterial strains that are best suited to the new circumstances. Thus, although we sometimes talk of a certain species "developing" resistance to a drug, we can see that resistance usually *doesn't* "develop" after the fact; it's existed all along but simply hasn't been expressed.

This scenario is complicated by the fact that microbes can, under certain circumstances, transfer resistance to other members of their species, and even to *other* types of species. Resistance to penicillin comes from a substance called *penicillinase*, which chemically breaks the drug down into components that are harmless to pathogens. The ability to create penicillinase comes from a specific gene that is passed on to a cell's offspring when it divides. But sometimes a cell will come across a free-floating gene from another bacterium and take it for itself, thereby gaining that gene's activity. Sometimes other cells intervene and carry the gene from one bacterium to another. And sometimes, by means of a complex interaction called *conjugation,* bacteria exchange this material with each other directly. Thus, a penicillin-resistant specimen of the normally friendly *E. coli* might pass along resistance to a virulent pathogen. Even more unfortunate, conjugation can simultaneously transfer resistance to a variety of drugs, and can confer even greater resistance than that possessed by the microbe from which the gene originally came.

No matter how a species gains resistance, the drama unfolds the same way. A drug scores victory after victory at first, all the while encouraging the spread of resistant strains. In the end, then, the drug becomes its own worst enemy by creating an environment in which resistant microbes flourish.

Now, this isn't to suggest that penicillin or any of the other antibiotics are on the verge of becoming obsolete. In the first place, many types of pathogens never become resistant. Also, the use of antibiotics isn't, as a rule, so widespread that it affects the entire world population of any particular microbe. In other words, if we think of penicillin as a plague among bacteria, we can see that it's a very localized one, largely confined to hospitals. (In fact, antibiotics are used so much in hospitals, there's no better breeding ground for antibiotic-resistant microbes. For that reason, doctors have all but abandoned the use of ordinary penicillin for the treatment of "nosocomial"—that is, hospital-acquired—infections.)

Another means of combating resistance is to use other types of antibiotics, which is exactly what is done for nosocomial infections. Although microbes resistant to, say, penicillin are often resistant to other, related compounds, there are usually enough variations to outsmart even the most tenacious bugs. Thus, for penicillin-resistant infections, a doctor might prescribe such antibiotics as erythromycin or tetracycline, which are chemically distinct from penicillin.

But, you ask, won't at least some of these microbes eventually prove resistant to these other drugs as well? The answer, unfortunately, is yes. To a certain extent, we're involved in a cat-and-mouse game with our ancient microbial enemies, as every new advance brings with it the possibility of even more resistant organisms. The advances of the last half century have been impressive—amazing, even—and the array of powerful antibiotics can be expected to control bacterial infections for the foreseeable future. But the key word here is *control,* not eradicate; most pathogens will, in all likelihood, always be with us.

There were two major reasons why the discovery of penicillin marked the beginning and not the end of the story of antibiotics. One was this problem of resistance, which spurred researchers to continue to look for new antibiotics. A more immediate reason, though, was the fact that penicillin, as we've seen, isn't effective against all types of bacteria. Fleming himself was the first to realize this, as his early studies in Petri dishes showed that the penicillium mold killed only certain types of bacteria.

The story of antibiotics continues with René Dubos, whose interest lay not in Petri dishes but in the soil. Dubos was intrigued by a phenomenon first noted by Pasteur. While studying anthrax, a disease that attacks livestock, Pasteur noted that sheep could safely graze in fields where anthrax-ridden carcasses had been buried. Why, he asked, didn't they sicken and die from their contact with the infected soil? Had the anthrax germs disappeared from the soil, and if so, how? In fact, what happened to *all* the pathogens in buried corpses? Why wasn't the entire world a vast cesspool of killer pathogens? Was there something in the earth that prevented their spread?

Pasteur theorized that indeed there was, and to prove it he mixed living anthrax-producing organisms with ordinary soil. The result, just as he suspected, was that the anthrax germs were destroyed.

Wonder Drugs That Weren't: Sulfanilamide Elixir

Before the discovery of penicillin, the only class of drugs that had any effectiveness against bacterial infections were the sulfa drugs, which therefore enjoyed a great deal of popularity. In 1937, the Tennessee firm of Massengill and Company introduced a liquid form of sulfanilamide, apparently believing that Southerners preferred syrups to pills when it was time to take their medicine. They found that sulfanilamide would not dissolve in alcohol or water, so instead a Massengill chemist used diethylene glycol as the solvent.

Unfortunately, U.S. drug laws in 1938 required only that drugs brought to the marketplace be properly labeled; it required no testing for effectiveness or even safety in humans. Massengill conformed to the letter of the law; it performed no animal or human tests on its "Elixir Sulfanilamide" before offering it for sale. Even worse, it refused to disclose the ingredients of the elixir, claiming that the formula was a trade secret. But had Massengill tested diethylene glycol in animal studies, it would have learned that the chemical causes slow, agonizing death by destroying the kidneys.

Shortly after the drug was marketed, the American Medical Association received a telegram from Tulsa, Oklahoma. AMA President Dr. Morris Fishbein learned from the telegram that six people in Tulsa had died of kidney failure after taking Elixir Sulfanilamide. Dr. Fishbein contacted Massengill and, after much prodding, learned that the solvent was toxic diethylene glycol.

Once notified, the FDA acted quickly to seize the Elixir. Warnings were issued via newspapers, radio stations, and posters. Even so, the Elixir Sulfanilamide claimed at least 108 victims, including the Massengill chemist who created it, who committed suicide.

Because U.S. drug laws did not require a drug to be tested for safety before it was marketed, the FDA was forced to rely on a legal technicality to seize the drug. It had been "mislabeled," the FDA said, since an "elixir" was defined as a drug dissolved in alcohol.

A positive result of this tragedy was a strengthening of the FDA's authority. Public outrage forced Congress to pass the Food, Drug, and Cosmetic Act of 1938, which for the first time imposed the commonsense requirement that drugs be tested for toxicity before they were introduced. As "tough" as the new law was, it only required drugs to be safe; it said nothing about their efficacy. That failing would not be corrected for nearly 25 years, when the law was amended in the wake of the thalidomide tragedy.

This was but another example of his maxim, "Life hinders life." With this simple and elegant experiment, Pasteur planted the seed of an idea that Dubos and others would nurture: The earth is teeming with beneficial organisms—"police of the soil," as one writer terms them—that invade decaying carcasses and destroy the pathogens they find there.

Others had followed up on Pasteur's line of reasoning, and when Dubos began thinking about the problem in the 1920s, it was already well established that soil contained many organisms capable of destroying pathogenic bacteria. What Dubos wanted to do was to systematically search for pathogen-destroying organisms in samples of soil. After many years of other research, he was finally able, in 1937, to get these experiments under way. His approach was simple but elegant. He first collected soil samples from a variety of sources—gardens, dumps, fields, forests, peat bogs, swamps, quarries, and elsewhere— and placed each one in a flask. He waited until the microbes had used up all traces of food in the flask, and then added to each one a liberal portion of pneumococci.

Dubos left the flasks alone for nearly a year, permitting the pathogens and soil microbes to fight each other without interference. When he finally examined them, the experiment at first appeared to be a failure—none of the soil samples showed *any* sign of life.

Almost none, that is. In one, there flourished colonies of tiny rod-shaped bacteria—*Bacillus brevis,* as Dubos termed them—which had apparently destroyed the pneumococcal germs.

Dubos grew cultures of *B. brevis* and, when the cultures were extensive enough, he isolated the bacteria-killing substance they produced. When he tested it, he found that it killed staphylococci and streptococci as well as pneumococci.

Dubos called this miracle substance tyrothricin, and next he tried it in mice. First he infected the mice with pneumococci, and, once they'd come down with pneumonia, gave them shots of tyrothricin. Almost immediately, their condition improved: their lungs cleared, their fevers dropped, and they seemed fully recovered.

Then disaster struck. First one, then another mouse suddenly died; in the end, not a single one survived. Laboratory tests showed that the tyrothricin had destroyed the mice's red blood cells.

Like Fleming, who at about this same time had abandoned his research on penicillin, Dubos was on the verge of giving up. But doctors who were aware of his experiments assured him that he was throwing in the towel too soon. Perhaps, they suggested, the substance could be used *externally,* for skin infections, eye infections, and the like.

Spurred on by this possibility, Dubos continued his attempts to purify this antibacterial substance. He and his fellow researchers discovered that tyrothricin could be split into two components, gramicidin and tyrocidine, and that these were as effective as tyrothricin. Soon ointments containing these substances became commercially available and, just as the doctors had predicted, were immensely useful in treating external bacterial infections. They could, it was discovered, even be used in a mouthwash for oral infections; any that was swallowed was neutralized in the stomach and never entered the bloodstream.

One of these products—gramicidin—is still used today, although there now exist many other effective antibiotics for the treatment of external infections. But Dubos's contribution to the modern science—and business—of pharmacology extends far beyond the substances he discovered. As we will see, his *approach*—systematically testing soil samples for evidence of useful new drugs—would establish a pattern leading to the discovery of a host of new and useful drugs, from streptomycin to cyclosporine. In addition, his approach would shape the development of the pharmaceutical industry, which was, even as Dubos worked, emerging from the colorful and sordid days of snake-oil remedies to become the modern and highly technological enterprises that they are today.

The Next Great Advance: Streptomycin

Selman Waksman, a professor at Rutgers University in New Jersey and Dubos's former boss, shared with him an interest in the potential of substances within the earth to cure disease. In fact, Waksman and Dubos had together devised the experiments that, with much modification, led to the discovery of tyrothricin.

Unfortunately, the undertaking Waksman and his colleagues had set out for themselves proved to be even larger than they themselves had imagined, and before long they had more than 10,000 different cultures growing.

Waksman's particular interest lay in the fungus *Streptomyces griseus,* and he believed that it had great potential as a source of antibiotic drugs. But it was no easy task to study *S. griseus,* because it exhibits different properties virtually every time it's grown. This, in fact, was one reason Waksman was interested in the organism, since he hoped that among the many variants there would be at least one that would lead to a breakthrough.

A sick chicken then entered the picture. Rutgers University, where Waksman worked, was then, and is now, an important center of agricultural research, and for that reason a poultry breeder had brought an ailing hen to its Agricultural Research Station. During the examination of the bird a small white spot was found in her throat, which was subsequently found to be yet another variety of *S. griseus.*

Knowing of Waksman's experiments, workers at the research station turned over a sample of the material to the investigators, who started growing a larger sample of it. When they had enough to work with, they ran the usual tests and found that their five long years of work had at last paid off.

Tests of the substance produced by this strain of *S. griseus* showed that it was indeed effective against many pathogens. Unfortunately, there were also some potentially serious side effects, but even so, it promised to be an effective and important addition to the physician's arsenal against infection. At the same time it, along with tyrothricin, demonstrated that penicillin was not a fluke and that there were potentially many more sources of antibiotics, literally at our feet.

Waksman's team retrieved soil samples from the poultry breeder's yard, where they found more *S. griseus* capable of producing the life-saving substance. Further refinements finally led to a drug they named streptomycin.

Streptomycin was less toxic than the original extract from which it was developed, and further study showed it to kill an impressive array of pathogens. Doctors using the drug began to report remarkable successes. An outbreak of plague in India offered an opportunity to try it against that ancient scourge, and it reduced the epidemic's death rate from nearly 70 percent to 4 percent.

But most important was the drug's effectiveness against tuberculosis. Before streptomycin, tuberculosis had proved resistant to every drug that had been tried against it. Indeed, medicine had little to offer victims of this wasting and usually fatal disease other than admission to a sanatorium. (These sanatoria were the most popular means of treating tuberculosis in the late nineteenth and early twentieth century. Usually situated on wooded mountaintops or in the desert, they supposedly helped the patient recover by providing rest and unpolluted air. Although it's questionable whether they actually provided much help to their *patients,* they did help reduce the mortality rate from tuberculosis by isolating communicable cases from other healthy persons.)

Doctors first used streptomycin to treat tuberculosis at the Mayo Clinic in Rochester, Minnesota, late in 1944. The patient was a young woman who had already undergone an operation in which much of her right lung had been removed in an effort to stop the disease. Streptomycin cured her where surgery had failed—the first time that drugs had conquered this killer. Along with another antibiotic, isoniazid, that was discovered a few years later, streptomycin would go on to wipe out tuberculosis as a major killer.

But in spite of streptomycin's successes, the problem of side effects kept cropping up. Most were minor and temporary—inflammation where the drug was injected, skin rashes, fever, and low blood pressure—but some were much more serious. The drug affected hearing and could even cause deafness; it could also cause extreme dizziness and vision disturbances—sometimes even blindness.

Further research on the drug yielded preparations that were much purer than Waksman's extracts, but the side effects persisted. Doctors noticed that they were similar to the effects of a poison called guanidine, and when chemists determined the drug's chemistry, they found out why: it contained chemical structures that were closely related to those of guanidine.

Chemists tried removing these guanidine "groups," as they're called, from streptomycin, but they found them to be essential to its antibiotic activity. Finally, in 1953, they learned that the toxic effects could be greatly reduced by combining streptomycin with pantothenic acid, which is one of the B-complex vitamins. Tests of the new combination showed that it retained streptomycin's antibiotic potency, but that the symptoms of dizziness, nausea, and headaches disappeared. The hearing-loss problem was also greatly reduced.

Wonder Drugs That Weren't: Chloramphenicol

Chloramphenicol was first marketed in 1949 by Parke-Davis, and it quickly attained a reputation as a powerful and versatile antibiotic. Throughout the 1950s, doctors enthusiastically prescribed it for typhoid fever, hemophilus influenza, and many other kinds of infections. Spurred on by Parke-Davis's advertising campaigns, doctors also prescribed it (as they did many other antibiotics) needlessly for illnesses that were often trivial or unaffected by antibiotics.

Unfortunately, chloramphenicol had the potential for causing aplastic anemia, a condition in which the body becomes unable to manufacture red blood cells. This side effect was fairly rare, occurring in about one patient in 25,000 to 40,000. However, when it did occur, it was fatal.

Because of chloramphenicol's unquestioned—and continuing—value in certain serious infections, the FDA decided not to take it off the market, but it did caution physicians that they should prescribe it only when absolutely necessary.

After this announcement, prescription sales for chloramphenicol did drop off—for a while. Soon, however, Parke-Davis had mounted a campaign that clouded the FDA's clear-cut recommendation. The company's promotional material claimed that the FDA warning actually constituted an *endorsement* of the drug, and that it was "undoubtedly the highest compliment ever handed the medical staff of our company." In other statements concerning publicity over the FDA action, Parke-Davis referred to "the unethical tactics being employed by representatives of certain competitors" and denounced the popular press for "careless or illogical deductions, lack of scientific understanding, use of material out of context, and lack of proper perspective." Parke-Davis representatives were told not to bring up the question of toxicity "unless the physician brings up the subject."

By 1964, chloramphenicol was being prescribed for more than 3.5 million patients a year. More than 90 percent of them received it unnecessarily—despite the fact that the drug's dangers supposedly had been well known for 15 years. In all, it's estimated that several hundred people died in the United States as a result. The popularity of chloramphenicol began to drop only after congressional hearings focused on the drug in 1967, during which evidence came to light about Parke-Davis's promotional techniques and the dangers of chloramphenicol first became widely known to consumers.

Streptomycin Today

The discovery of streptomycin created a new class of antibiotic drugs, the aminoglycosides. Other members of this class, all chemically related to streptomycin, include such drugs as neomycin, kanamycin, and gentamicin.

These newer members of the family are often more effective or less toxic—or both—than streptomycin itself, and for that reason Waksman's original wonder drug isn't used much anymore. But the aminoglycosides as a group *are* important and are the drugs of choice against bacteria whose cell walls are unaffected by penicillin. Though effective, the drugs share streptomycin's drawbacks—prolonged use still can cause nerve damage and hearing loss as well as damage to the kidneys—and for these reasons doctors use them only for the treatment of serious infections. In addition, many organisms have become totally resistant to streptomycin and the other aminoglycosides, which further limits their usefulness.

But just as with Dubos's tyrothricin, streptomycin's place in the history of pharmaceuticals is secure. Its discovery complemented penicillin's—both because it acted against penicillin-resistant organisms and because it pointed the way toward discovery of even more effective antibiotics. By demonstrating the fact that penicillin was not the only antibiotic to be found, it qualifies not merely as a wonder drug but as a true miracle drug—that is, one that substantially expands the horizons of medicine.

And, as we shall see in the next section, it was a watershed in medicine for another reason. After streptomycin, the discovery of new drugs largely became a matter of economics rather than luck.

The Search Continues

There is in the stories of penicillin, tyrothricin, and streptomycin a definite progression in the search for protection against harmful bacteria. Fleming happened across penicillin by accident, while Dubos and Waksman, realizing the broader implications of Fleming's discovery, set out to search systematically for antibiotic-producing organisms.

Waksman's experiments, in particular, proved two things: first, that this systematic approach could indeed lead to new antibiotics, and second, that it was an enormously expensive and time-consuming process.

The pharmaceutical companies of the day were aware of this, but they also sensed that the financial reward would be equally great for any firm that discovered new and improved antibiotics.

And so, taking their cue from Dubos and Waksman, they began to set up extensive research projects of their own. The concept was the same; only the scale was different. Lederle Laboratories, for example, asked every employee, every friend, every acquaintance, to bring them soil samples. Their botanists brought in samples from farms, forests, gardens, and meadows; others brought samples collected on travels throughout the world. The company sent letters around the world requesting more samples; each one contained a small shovel and several bags. Week after week the samples came into the company's headquarters in Pearl River, New York, and in the end, researchers had more than 800 samples from around the world.

A hundred researchers, under the direction of botanist Benjamin Duggar, now started the massive task of sorting through all this raw material. Each sample went into a jug of water, which was shaken for an hour. The resulting mud was then added to a flask containing nutrients for the microbes in the samples to feed on.

A few days later, the flasks were filled with weblike colonies of microbes. The contents were carefully registered, with special attention being given to new or unfamiliar organisms.

Next, samples of these organisms were introduced into colonies of pathogens, and the waiting began anew. In most cases, nothing happened, but now and then a fungus appeared that inhibited the growth of the bacteria. When this happened, the researchers would either store the responsible fungus in a lump of sterile soil or, if it looked especially promising, would continue to test its antibiotic properties.

From the 800 soil samples, Duggar occasionally encountered a bright yellow fungus that, he learned, was especially effective at killing pathogens. He called the fungus *Streptomyces aureofaciens*. The last half of the name is Latin for "gold-making"; Duggar was referring to its golden color, but the mold would eventually make gold of a decidedly different kind for Lederle Laboratories. From it, researchers eventually developed a drug they called Aureomycin® (chlortetracycline), which was effective not only against penicillin-sensitive organisms but against a range of others as well.

Soon, another pharmaceutical company, Charles Pfizer & Co., got into the act on an even larger scale. Whereas Duggar had worked with 800 soil samples at Lederle, Pfizer researchers started with 116,000. Using the same techniques as Duggar, they did indeed find antibiotics. They found streptomycin, for example, and gramicidin. They even found chlortetracycline. But, of course, none of these "discoveries" had any commercial value, since they didn't represent anything new.

Finally, after spending millions of dollars, the Pfizer team did discover a new antibiotic. They called it Terramycin® (oxytetracycline) after the Latin for earth and found that it, like Aureomycin®, was a powerful broad-spectrum antibiotic.

Further studies revealed that the new drug was chemically very similar to Aureomycin®, and that both were in fact complicated versions of a substance called *tetracycline*—whose existence was only theoretical at the time. Upon publication of these studies, researchers at both Pfizer and Lederle set out to create pure tetracycline. The race ended in a tie, as both firms published the results of their work in the same issue of the *Journal of the American Chemical Society*.

After Tetracycline: Modest Advances

Since the days of Fleming, Waksman, and Duggar, the story of antibiotics has mostly been one of small improvements rather than astounding breakthroughs. Researchers have discovered dozens of new antibiotics in the past thirty-odd years, but the mainstays of therapy against bacterial infections remain the penicillin group, the aminoglycosides, and the tetracyclines.

Where these don't work or can't be used, doctors have some other options. The *cephalosporins*, for example, which were originally isolated from an organism living near a sewer outlet on the coast of Italy, have effects similar to those of penicillin. *Erythromycin*, which came from a Philippine soil sample, is often used in cases where allergies or resistance prevent the use of penicillin. But even so, Fleming's original discovery is still prescribed more than any other antibiotic.

* * *

We've witnessed in this chapter a remarkable progression from Alexander Fleming's solitary experiments to the massive undertakings that led to the discovery of the tetracyclines and other modern antibiotics—a series of events that revolutionized medicine more than all of the other discoveries since Hippocrates. Suddenly, in less than a lifetime, the role of the physician has profoundly changed. No longer the simple minister of the flesh, whose most effective tools were sympathy and a deep appreciation of the body's ability to heal itself, modern physicians must orchestrate their patients' care with all the finesse of a musical conductor and must have intimate knowledge of such basic scientific fields as chemistry, physics, and microbiology.

If the development of the antibiotics has made medicine more of a science, it has also made it more of a business. The success of Aureomycin® and the other tetracyclines in particular demonstrated that there was money to be made in the development of new and effective drugs. And, as we'll see in Chapter 9, the techniques used to discover the antibiotics are far from outmoded; they are, in fact, the foundation for some of the very latest breakthroughs in drug research. From Pasteur to Duggar, the visionary scientists of this era did their work well and charted a course that others would follow with equal success.

4

From Cowpox to Cancer: Vaccines and the Immune System

There's a special canister in a laboratory in Atlanta, kept locked away under tight 24-hour security, with only a handful of scientists permitted to go near it. In Moscow there's a similar receptacle. Together they represent the last remnants of a microbial living fossil, an organism that has otherwise vanished from the face of the earth. This tiny creature, which once roamed the earth, succumbed neither to changing climates nor the encroachment of civilization; it was hunted into extinction.

Through desert and jungle, across vast oceans and icy plains, with the cooperation of virtually every civilized government on the planet, scientists tracked this tiny virus like a pack of hounds on the trail of a fox.

And now, left with only these two remaining colonies, American and Soviet scientists are faced with a Godlike decision. Should they preserve the samples for study by future generations of scientists? Or should they destroy them and close the book forever on the greatest scourge mankind has ever known—a plague that has over countless centuries killed billions of human beings, and even now can only be prevented, not cured? If they kill the colonies, it will mark the first time that mankind has intentionally obliterated an entire species.

It will mark the end of smallpox.

Though few would note the passing of smallpox and none would lament it, its story is not an entirely evil one. It has, in fact, left behind a gift for mankind—a gift as precious as the disease itself is terrible. For out of the struggle to find protection from the dreaded pox came the first understanding—dim at first, and then more clear over succeeding generations—of how the body protects itself against disease. And now, even as smallpox is on the brink of disappearing from the memory of man, this legacy promises new therapy for everything from tooth decay to cancer.

Smallpox: Biography of a Killer

Originally native to the Middle East, smallpox was brought to Europe by the returning armies of the Crusades. Once there, it quickly established itself as the continent's number-one killer, taking even more lives than the Black Death. In England during the seventeenth century, one person in four could look forward to death by smallpox, and virtually no one escaped the disfiguring pockmarks left by the disease. During the eighteenth century, some 60 million people—20 times the population of the newly created United States—succumbed to the disease in Europe alone.

Among the natives of the New World, smallpox wreaked havoc on a scale that today is associated only with nuclear war. In many communities more than half the inhabitants died in a matter of weeks—an orgy of death that did more than the conquistadors and their firearms to hasten the collapse of resistance to the European invaders.

From the Eskimo villages of Alaska to the jungles of Guatemala, on down to Tierra del Fuego at the very tip of South America, the white man spread his deadly gift from beyond the sea. Sometimes it was done intentionally; British soldiers, for instance, received the following instruction: "You will do well to try to inoculate the Indians by means of blankets as well as to try every other method that can serve to extirpate this execrable race."

The first step toward loosening the worldwide stranglehold of smallpox came from an unlikely source: a British aristocrat by the name of Lady Mary Wortley Montagu. Uncharacteristically liberated for a lady of the sixteenth-century English aristocracy, she was by all accounts as beautiful as she was unconventional. At nineteen she eloped with Wortley Montagu, who later became Britain's ambassador to Turkey; as the ambassador's wife, she donned disguises and roamed through parts of Constantinople that were not considered suitable for a young English lady of taste and refinement.

It was on one of these excursions that she observed a peculiar practice, later recounted in a letter to a friend:

> Apropos of distempers I am going to tell you a thing that I am sure will make you wish yourself here. The smallpox, so fatal, and so general among us, is here entirely harmless by the invention of *ingrafting,* which is the name they give it. There is a set of old women who make it their business to perform the operation every autumn in the month of September, when the great heat is abated. People send to one another to know if any of their family has a mind to have the smallpox; they make parties for this purpose and when they are met (commonly fifteen or sixteen together) the old woman comes with a nut-shell full of the matter of the best small-pox and asks you what veins you please to have opened. She immediately rips open that you offer her with a large needle (which gives you no more pain than a common scratch) and puts into the vein as much venom as can be upon the head of her needle, and after binds up the little wound with a hollow bit of shell; and in this way opens up four or five veins. . . . The children or young patients play together all the rest of the day, and are in perfect health to the eighth. Then the fever begins to seize them, and they keep their beds two days, very seldom three. They have very rarely above twenty or thirty [pocks] in their faces, which never mark; and in eight days' time they are as well as before their illness.

Thus was the Western world first exposed to the idea of vaccination through the keen eye of Lady Mary Wortley Montagu. This idea made perfect sense, for everyone knew that persons who once survived smallpox never got it again. So why not get the disease when you were young, healthy, and most likely to recover? Thus, Lady Mary fully expected the British medical community to welcome her discovery with open arms. But, to her surprise, when she sought to introduce the practice in England, condemnation was swift and severe. Outrageous! puffed the learned professors of medicine; the barbarous proposal would destroy the youth of the kingdom. Blasphemous!

thundered the clergy; how dare man attempt to intervene in a fate ordained by God? Shocking! cried the papers; what mother would risk the lives of her children so foolishly?

Like many good ideas, this one cut across the grain of conventional wisdom and was rejected out of hand by those who should have been most qualified to see its virtues. And yet even on such barren ground, the idea took root, nourished by the fears and hopes of a population under siege. Ignoring the wisdom of the professors, a layman named Robert Sutton opened a vaccination center in Essex with the help of his two sons. Common people, oblivious to the dire warnings of the physicians, clergy, and newspapers, flocked to Sutton's center. Eventually, Sutton and his sons vaccinated more than 17,000 people—only five of whom died.

Still the idea met with resistance. In America, Cotton Mather of Massachusetts took on the role that Lady Mary had played in Britain—with about as much luck. Someone threw a bomb into his window, and an angry mob attacked Dr. Zabdiel Boylston, a Boston physician who had also publicly supported vaccination. In time, however, cooler heads prevailed, and the practice at last came to be accepted by physicians and the community at large.

Principles of Vaccination

These early methods illustrate the first principle of vaccination: (1) Infection with certain kinds of diseases creates immunity from later reinfection. Often, as with smallpox, the immunity is lifelong, but in other cases immunity may fade after a time (hence the need for "booster" shots for, say, tetanus). Even a common cold renders you immune from the responsible virus for a brief period of time (typically a few weeks); you may have noticed that you only catch a cold once when it's going around.

But a second principle of vaccination—one that greatly expanded the potential for preventing all sorts of dread diseases—did not become apparent until the end of the 1700s, when Edward Jenner publicized the results of his experiments with cowpox. Jenner, an English physician from the dairy-farming region of Gloucestershire, was aware of the widespread belief among the people of the region that cowpox, a mild disease contracted from cows, provided immunity against smallpox. To test this idea, Jenner first exposed a young boy to cowpox and a month or two later inoculated him with smallpox. (The experiment sounds risky, but by Jenner's day smallpox inoculation was accepted practice for creating immunity.) Just as Jenner suspected, the boy showed no signs whatsoever of smallpox.

Jenner's discovery had vast practical significance, for it meant that people could be vaccinated against smallpox by exposure to a disease no more serious than chickenpox or the flu. But of even greater significance in the long run was that he'd established the second principle of vaccination: (2) One could be vaccinated against a disease without being exposed to the disease itself.

Jenner's technique came in for some ridicule at first—an engraving of the day shows his patients with cows growing from the vaccination sites on their arms—but it quickly became popular. The simple country doctor became a hero, the British Parliament voted to give him a prize of 10,000 British pounds, and the king rewarded him with a knighthood.

Even today 10,000 pounds is a fair amount of money; in Jenner's day it was a fortune. But for the newly knighted Edward, it was a source of tribulation, for soon it came to light that he had not been the first to use the cowpox vaccination. Twenty years before Jenner's first experiment, a farmer by the name of Benjamin Jesty had used a stocking needle to scratch cowpox material into the arms of his wife and children. Just as Jenner would do 20 years later, Jesty then inoculated his "patients" with smallpox, and found that they were totally immune. After this brief excursion into medicine, Jesty returned once more to his farming. When, 20 years later, he heard of Jenner and the 10,000 pounds, he got in touch with his local Member of Parliament to lodge a protest.

Unfortunately, Jesty received neither 10,000 pounds nor a knighthood. He was invited to London, where he had his portrait painted and received a pair of gold-mounted needles as a souvenir of his contribution to medicine. From there he presumably returned to his farm, where he could contemplate in idle moments upon the fact that it does indeed pay to advertise.

Further Work on Vaccines

Jesty might have consoled himself with the fact that the fame that eluded him didn't sit too well with Jenner. He was no sophisticate, and he soon left London for the simpler life of

Gloucestershire. Perhaps he also felt himself to be something of a fraud, for he reportedly suffered great disappointment and embarrassment over the fact that he couldn't explain why his great discovery worked.

But he needn't have felt badly, for he lacked an essential piece of the puzzle. It was not until Louis Pasteur formulated his germ theory of disease in the nineteenth century that anyone would begin to understand the workings of such diseases as smallpox, and no progress would occur in the area of vaccines for half a century.

Pasteur himself developed vaccines against anthrax (a disease of cattle) and rabies, and in so doing discovered a third great principle of immunization: (3) immunization could be created by exposure to a weakened form of the infectious organism. He prepared a vaccine from the spinal cord of a rabbit who had died from rabies and used it successfully to immunize dogs. He began with a vaccine prepared from a 14-day-old cord, followed by one from a 13-day-old cord and so on until fresh cord could be used. After this series of injections, the dogs in his experiments were immune to rabies.

Pasteur had reservations about using the rabies vaccine on humans, until one day when a young boy named Joseph Meister was brought to him. Joseph had been bitten by a rabid dog, and was certain to die if he was not treated. With nothing to lose, Pasteur agreed to try the new rabies vaccine. Over the next several days, the boy received a series of 13 injections, while Pasteur himself, hanging between hope and dread, suffered from nightmares and was unable to work.

But despite all his doubts, the vaccine did work, and young Joseph Meister became the first known survivor of rabies. He returned to his home in the Alsace region of France; years later he became the gatekeeper at the Pasteur Institute in Paris.

The Immune System: A Primer

Despite the vaccine's success, Pasteur knew little more than Jenner about what was actually occurring in his patient's body. He knew only what everyone in his time knew—that exposure to some diseases created immunity against later infection—and he guessed that exposure to a weakened form of the disease might also trigger an immune response without putting the patient at risk.

He was, of course, right. But this is as far as his understanding went. Pasteur's genius lay in his ability to make great mental leaps, guided by nothing more than careful observation and shrewd intuition; as a result, he often came up with practical solutions before he had a theory to explain them. Only later would researchers begin to discover *why* his guesses about vaccines for anthrax and rabies had been correct.

In the years since Pasteur, researchers have learned a great deal about the immune system and how it works, and have discovered it to be one of the most fascinating and complex topics in all the world of medicine. And although they have long since solved the puzzle that confounded Jenner and Pasteur, along the way they've discovered the immune system has far more mysteries than those two pioneers ever suspected.

As we saw in the chapter on antibiotics, the human body has some very effective defenses against outsiders. The skin, like China's Great Wall, forms a nearly seamless physical barrier that repels foreign invaders. If, say, a band of smallpox viruses somehow penetrated this first obstacle, it would be met by one-celled sentries, who would engage it in battle and call for reinforcements.

Now the body does something truly magical. Even as these cells (called *lymphocytes*) attack the virus, they are studying it. Like the British plane spotters of World War II who learned the silhouettes of German bombers so that they could warn the RAF of enemy raids, the lymphocytes learn to recognize the chemical "silhouettes"—or *antigens,* as they're known to biologists—of the invading bacteria or viruses. Once they've absorbed this information, the lymphocytes can manufacture custom-designed chemicals (proteins known as *antibodies*) that attach themselves to the invaders and either destroy them directly or help other sentry cells identify and finish them off.

But it may take a week or longer for this process to occur—time in which a person's life may be hanging in the balance. If the body is strong and otherwise healthy, it can vigorously resist the invader during this critical time; if it is old, malnourished, or otherwise debilitated—or if the infection is simply too overwhelming—the victim may die before the immune system has a chance to prevail.

If the smallpox virus is successfully repelled, yet another wondrous thing happens. The immune system somehow stores the smallpox "silhouette," and if ever new smallpox viruses were to invade—whether 6 hours later or 60 years later—

smallpox antibodies would already be on the scene, ready to destroy the invaders before they could establish a beachhead.

By now you may have guessed what Jenner and Pasteur could not know—that the cowpox vaccine worked because cowpox and smallpox have similar antigens. Thus, when the body is infected with the relatively benign cowpox virus, the lymphocytes manufacture antibodies that are also effective against its dreaded cousin, smallpox.

This elegant system, of course, furnishes the explanation not only for Jenner's discovery, but also for the ingrafting method observed by Lady Mary Wortley Montagu in Constantinople and later adopted in Europe and America. It also explains Pasteur's success against rabies. His series of inoculations, beginning with a preparation of nearly dead virus, stimulated production of antibodies without actually bringing on the disease itself. (Incidentally, rabies is one of the few diseases for which vaccination can be initiated *after* exposure; the reason is the disease's exceptionally long *incubation period*—that is, the time between exposure and actual onset of the disease.)

Scientists call the process we've looked at thus far *active immunity,* since the body actively manufactures antibodies. There is, in addition, another type of immunity—*passive immunity*. It's a sort of pharmacological shortcut to protection and consists of supplying other people's antibodies to a patient who does not have or cannot manufacture his own.

For many years this basic picture governed our understanding of the immune system and our ability to manipulate it. New vaccines, such as those for polio, mumps, and measles, generally were developed along the lines of Pasteur's rabies vaccine, with the use of dead or altered organisms intended to provoke the immune system into forming antibodies. But the process is a difficult and risky one, and success owes as much to luck as to anything else. As a result, only a relative handful of vaccines have been developed, and many diseases for which vaccines are theoretically possible remain untamed. Today, however, a number of new discoveries have already begun to change that picture, providing us with more new vaccines over the past few years than at any time since the days of Jenner. And this is only the beginning. More vaccines are in the works, and researchers believe that vaccines for everything from tooth decay to AIDS may lie just over the horizon.

The Quest for "Magic Bullets"

For years doctors have dreamed of "magic bullets"—drugs that would seek out and destroy disease and yet leave the rest of the body untouched. To doctors of the early 20th century, the idea seemed little more than science fiction—a fantasy with no practical utility—until the discovery of penicillin. Faced with that momentous event, doctors and researchers suddenly had to come to grips with the fact that magic bullets not only were possible, but actually existed—a realization that revolutionized the very foundations of medicine.

The search for magic bullets did not end with antibiotics, however. Today it has led to the field of immunology, where researchers are now feeling much the same excitement that the discoverers of antibiotics experienced half a century ago. Indeed, recent discoveries have opened up the possibility of not just new bullets, but entire new arsenals of drugs.

These discoveries are part of the new field of genetic engineering. Just 15 years ago, the idea of being able to alter at will the biological blueprint of living things seemed as far-fetched as, say, desktop computers. And yet genetic engineering not only exists, but has already moved into the world of commerce.

Genetic engineering is sometimes referred to, half-jokingly, as the stitching together of "designer genes"—a description that's not far off the mark. Genes serve as biochemical instruction manuals for every living thing, from amoebas to palm trees to monkeys to people.

All of this is really nothing more than ninth-grade biology, but until very recently it represented just about all that scientists knew about genes. Though they understood in general terms *how* genetics worked, they found it quite impossible to *predict* genetic results in any given case, much less *control* the process itself.

Not, that is, until the late 1970s, when researchers developed sophisticated methods for transferring genes from one organism to another. With this breakthrough, whole new possibilities suddenly emerged for treating genetic disorders. These possibilities are swiftly moving toward reality; for example, doctors are now investigating the possibility of treating genetic bone-marrow diseases by inserting the missing gene into the patient's own marrow cells, rather than doing bone marrow transplants from a donor.

But scientists have already created something that in its own way is even more spectacular: *entirely new forms of life* never seen in nature and custom-designed for specific purposes.

Let's return to the world of immunology for a true-life example. A few years ago, researchers at Merck Sharp & Dohme developed a powerful new vaccine against hepatitis B, a serious disease that afflicts millions of people worldwide and can cause liver disease and cancer. They made the vaccine by using antigens harvested from the blood of people who are carriers of the virus, and thus far its use has been limited by its high cost and the difficulty of recovering the antigens from the blood of carriers. Now, however, researchers at Merck and elsewhere have created a new, abundant source of hepatitis B antigen. They've identified the gene that controls the manufacture of the antigen and transferred it into yeast cells. The result is a new type of yeast with the curious ability to manufacture hepatitis B antigen. Vaccine derived from this yeast-produced antigen has already been tested in monkeys and found to be as effective as the original vaccine; a yeast-derived vaccine for humans is expected soon.

Much the same techniques are used to produce other substances that hold great therapeutic promise but which in the past have been too rare or too difficult to obtain. Many of these are substances produced within the body in minute amounts—for instance, t-PA (discussed in Chapter 5) and human growth hormone, a vital substance that governs normal growth and development and can prevent some kinds of dwarfism.

Monoclonal Antibodies—The Modern Magic Bullet

But perhaps the greatest potential for developing wondrous new drugs involves the use of genetic engineering techniques to combine cancer cells with antibody-secreting cells, forming new cells with characteristics of both. These *hybridomas* harness the high metabolic rate of cancer cells to produce large quantities of very pure antibodies—*monoclonal antibodies*—that seek out certain types of disease cells with great precision. Many scientists believe that monoclonal antibodies may prove to be the ultimate magic bullet.

So far, monoclonal antibodies have seen use mainly as a diagnostic tool exploiting their ability to bind to specific antigens to provide a rapid and accurate means of identifying disease-causing organisms. But their potential is vastly greater, and research is going full tilt. Recently, for instance, Johnson & Johnson sought approval from the U. S. Food and Drug Administration to begin marketing the first monoclonal antibody for use in humans—a preparation designed to block white blood cells that attack transplanted organs.

And this is only the beginning. Across the board, basic research on the frontiers of immunology is unearthing new discoveries so fast that the drug companies can hardly keep up. As a result, we're discovering that the immune system plays a role in a whole array of diseases that have long mystified physicians.

For instance, we now know that multiple sclerosis is caused by a defect in the immune system. In multiple sclerosis and myasthenia gravis, renegade antibodies attach themselves to nerve cells and provoke their destruction by white blood cells. Evidence is mounting that at least some forms of diabetes are also *autoimmune* diseases—that is, diseases in which the body is attacked by its own immune system—with the victims being the cells in the pancreas that manufacture the body's supply of insulin. All of these diseases are potentially treatable with custom-designed monoclonal antibodies.

But of all the news from the world of immunology, the most exciting is the progress we're making against cancer. New discoveries about why cancer occurs—and how it might be stopped—have suddenly put cancer specialists and immunologists on common ground. In fact, it's becoming increasingly clear that cancer is in many respects an immunological disorder. Like diabetes, it results from the body's own cells going berserk; like infection, it is often caused by external agents and is subject to control by the immune system. There are other links as well. It's no accident, for example, that persons whose immune systems are destroyed by the AIDS virus often develop an otherwise rare form of cancer known as Kaposi's sarcoma.

Armed with this newfound knowledge, cancer researchers are today more optimistic than ever. In fact, scientists who just a few years ago were cautioning that breakthroughs in cancer therapy were at least decades away now speak of new cures.

Already this knowledge is moving out of the laboratory and into clinical trials, and results are promising. Monoclonal antibodies have already proven to be important tools for the diagnosis of cancer, and clinical trials show them to be promising in their treatment as well. As a result, more and more researchers believe that cancer may, in the not-so-distant future, go the way of tuberculosis and polio—a fading bad memory to future generations.

The "War on Cancer": The Tide Begins to Turn

But haven't we heard all this before? The Nixon Administration, for example, provided millions of dollars of federal funds for cancer research, as optimistic scientists declared a "war on cancer" and suggested that they might be able to come up with a cure as a Bicentennial birthday present. And since then, there has been report after report of new breakthroughs and possibilities: cancer was caused by viruses, some reported; no, said others, it was an autoimmune disorder. The Bicentennial came and went; and still cancer took its awful toll. Interferon was touted as a possible magic bullet against cancer, but has failed to live up to its early overenthusiastic billing. For many types of cancer, the death rates are actually rising, not falling. Thus, it's no surprise that reports of new breakthroughs are met with raised eyebrows.

But, in fact, the fight against cancer has been a victim of poor public relations. Doctors have in fact made significant strides against many forms of cancer. Children who suffer from acute lymphoblastic leukemia, for example, have a five-year mortality rate of approximately 50 percent—a horrendous figure, until you realize that twenty years ago the survival rate was virtually nil. Similarly, Hodgkin's disease, a cancer that affects the body's lymph glands, was once considered incurable; today, 78 percent of its victims are alive five years after diagnosis. (The five-year survival rate is the benchmark used by scientists to determine the success of cancer treatment. Admittedly an arbitrary figure, it's used because there's no suitable way of determining when a patient is "cured" of cancer.) Melanoma (a malignant form of skin cancer), thyroid cancer, testicular cancer, and cancer of the endometrium all now have five-year survival rates of 80 percent or more.

A number of other factors besides drugs play a part in this progress. Prevention is a big factor—the success against melanoma, for instance, is largely due to the fact that its victims are getting to the doctor sooner, before the cancer has spread to other parts of the body. In addition, there have been advances in the treatment of cancer by surgery and radiation, and in methods of detecting cancer at earlier and more curable stages.

But the advances that doctors have achieved thus far with drug therapy have been impressive as well—especially considering the fine line that doctors must walk between helping and harming the patient. Anticancer drugs can cause severe and unpleasant side effects—vomiting, hair loss, and damage to the immune system, to name a few. Ironically, they can even cause cancer.

The reason these drugs are so toxic to humans is simple. Cancer cells arise from normal body cells, and there's not a lot of difference between the two. This makes it very difficult to find substances that can destroy one without harming the other. Penicillin, by contrast, works by taking advantage of differences in the cell walls of bacteria and body cells (see Chapter 3).

There is a major difference between cancer cells and most types of normal cells: the rate at which they grow and reproduce. This difference is exploited by conventional anticancer drugs, such as nitrogen mustard and cisplatin, which kill cells that are in the process of dividing. Since cancer cells divide more quickly than most normal cells, they're simply killed off at a faster rate.

If you think this approach lacks subtlety, you're right. First, it means that any normal cells that divide rapidly, such as bone marrow cells or hair follicles, will die in great numbers. This accounts for many of the side effects of anticancer drugs. But these cells are not the only victims, for nearly all the body's cells divide at a greater or lesser rate. Thus, these drugs are potent poisons, and the trick in using them is to destroy the disease without killing the patient.

As if all this weren't bad enough, this crude approach has to be 100 percent effective against the cancer cells; unlike pathogens, stray cancer cells won't likely be caught by the body's immune system. The immune system itself is reeling under the onslaught of the drugs; besides, the cancer has already proven that it can fend off attacks from the immune system.

And, to make matters worse, the cancer cells themselves have a few tricks up their sleeves. They possess an almost diabolical ability to develop resistance to the drugs. And they sometimes taper off their growth rate for a while, rendering the drugs relatively ineffective.

In light of all these drawbacks, it is perhaps a miracle that these drugs work at all, but, in their own sledgehammer way, they do. And through careful observation of their effects, doctors have come up with combinations of drugs that have slowly but surely chipped away at cancer's deadly toll.

The best results have come with cancers that are easily accessible to the drugs. For example, leukemia, a cancer of the white blood cells, is a better candidate for chemotherapy than, say, bone cancer, for the simple reason that leukemia cells are more likely to come into contact with the drugs as they both circulate through the bloodstream. In addition, it has become obvious that "cocktails," combinations of various anticancer drugs, usually work better than any of the drugs individually. Similarly, chemotherapy is sometimes combined with radiation therapy and surgery with results surpassing those of any of these methods used alone.

A Cure for Cancer?

But despite all these advances, cancer remains a fearsome killer, and the "war against cancer" has been so far a war of attrition. So why believe those optimists who say that we are at last on the verge of developing new cures?

For a number of reasons. First is the remarkable fact that scientists now understand on the most basic level how cancer occurs. They've discovered that certain genes, known as *oncogenes,* are responsible for many (and probably all) kinds of cancer. In normal cells, these genes are responsible for certain vital functions—most of them having to do with the growth and reproduction of the cell—but they're controlled by other genes that turn them on and off as necessary. Various agents—certain types of viruses, for example, or carcinogenic chemicals—can rearrange the cell's genes. If, as a result, an oncogene finds itself in a position where it is controlled by another type of gene known as a *promoter*, it begins to send out inappropriate chemical messages to the cell, instructing it to multiply wildly and grow in a rapid and disorganized fashion.

That is, if it gets the chance. The body ordinarily has some sophisticated defenses against these cancers-in-the-making. The cell has the ability to recognize foul-ups in the genetic code and repair them. Usually, no harm is done, unless the cell divides before repairs are complete. Only in that unlikely event are the flaws passed on to the cell's descendants.

But if the cells do inherit the defective gene, they're unable to recognize it as being flawed, and they become cancer cells. Even then, all is not lost. Researchers believe that the immune system almost always destroys such errant cells. Just how it does so and how it recognizes them are still mysteries. But the fact that the human body contains many trillions of cells implies that potentially cancerous cells arise with alarming frequency. The most curious thing about cancer is not that so many people get it, but that so many of us manage to avoid it for so long. Cancer is typically a disease of the elderly.

How does all this newfound insight translate into new therapy? Well, it hasn't just yet, but it provides clues as to how we might, for example, target drugs to cancerous cells with greater precision. By studying the oncogenes, scientists are learning just what sorts of chemical changes they cause in cells, and this knowledge in turn may enable pharmacologists to devise drugs that can recognize and home in on cancerous cells while bypassing normal ones.

Now, this work with oncogenes is still in the very early stages, but another avenue may lead to anticancer magic bullets even sooner. The heroes, again, are monoclonal antibodies. It turns out that many cancers possess distinctive antigens, and that it's possible to produce antibodies specifically targeted to those antigens. This knowledge has progressed far beyond the basic research stage; already it's been used to develop sensitive screening tests for various types of cancer, thus permitting earlier diagnosis and treatment.

The real hope of monoclonal antibodies, however, is not for diagnosis but for treatment. Clinical investigations are in the very earliest stages, and already results are promising. In one trial, 20 patients with intestinal cancer received varying doses of a specific monoclonal antibody; all had cancer that had metastasized, that is, spread to other parts of the body. The goal of the experiment was simply to determine whether the antibody was toxic to patients, yet even in this very preliminary study three patients were apparently cured.

These early studies have revealed some difficult problems that must be solved along the way. For example, it seems that tumors consist of multiple variants of cancer cells, each with their own set of antigens; thus, it's likely that therapy will require monoclonal-antibody "cocktails," that is, combinations of various specific antibodies similar to the "cocktails" of anticancer drugs.

Even then, it may be difficult to reach every individual cancer cell. Therefore, biochemists are looking at ways to attach antibodies to radioactive chemicals in such a way that the antibody kills not only the target cell, but the dozen or so cells immediately surrounding it. Since all the various cancer cells tend to cluster together, researchers hope that this method will kill all or most of the cancer cells while leaving the vast majority of normal body cells unscathed. Other investigations are attempting to link monoclonal antibodies with poisonous chemicals to achieve similar results.

Tumor Necrosis Factor

Genetic engineering has also opened up an entirely independent line of research by making available a substance known as *tumor necrosis factor* (TNF). Researchers at Memorial Sloan-Kettering Cancer Center first discovered this rare natural protein in 1975 and found that it apparently has the ability to destroy cancer cells while leaving normal cells unharmed. Tiny amounts of TNF are produced within the body, where it seems to play a role in our natural defenses against cancer, but until recently scientists weren't able to obtain enough TNF to study its potential as an anticancer agent.

But now at least four genetic-engineering companies around the world have independently developed TNF-producing microbes, opening the way for human testing to begin. In laboratory tests involving 62 different kinds of human cancer cells grown in the laboratory, TNF killed the cells in 19 cases, inhibited their growth in another 21, and had no effect on the remaining 22. If these figures hold up in human tests—and if TNF proves safe—scientists will have discovered the anticancer equivalent of penicillin.

What's Next?

Perhaps the most promising aspect of all of these discoveries is that there appear to be important links among all of them. It's as if scientists now have enough pieces of the puzzle in place that the big picture is beginning to emerge. The discovery of TNF, for example, explains a century-old mystery of cancer therapy, one first noted by surgeon William B. Coley. Coley discovered that some of his patients seemed to be cured of the disease after suffering a severe infection. Eventually it was learned that endotoxins, poisons produced by the invading bacteria, had a strong anticancer effect, but that they were too toxic to use in patients. Now it's known that the endotoxins help stimulate the body to produce TNF and that this is the source of their anticancer effects.

TNF is also linked with two other anticancer drugs that, until now, have failed to live up to their expectations. Interferon and the tuberculosis vaccine known as BCG both have some value as anticancer drugs, but neither has yielded the dramatic results that many scientists predicted for them. Recent research has revealed, however, that TNF and interferon together are much more effective than either used alone. It's also known that BCG, along with endotoxins, can stimulate the production of TNF within the body, a finding that may partially explain BCG's anticancer properties.

Where all of this seems to be leading is not so much to a single magic bullet as to a magic arsenal. Cancer therapy may one day combine monoclonal antibodies, TNF, interferon, BCG, anticancer vaccines, and other drugs only hinted at by current research. Traditional cancer drugs will undoubtedly continue to play a major role, as will radiation, surgery, and preventive efforts. Perhaps, with all these new and old tools, the greatest medical success story of the twentieth century may yet be the conquest of cancer.

5

Heartfelt Wonders: Cardiovascular Drugs

We Americans are living in the midst of a terrible epidemic: an epidemic of heart disease. Every year failing hearts kill more people than cancer, car accidents, infections, or any other cause—in fact, they account for half of all deaths recorded annually.

And yet strangely, it's an epidemic of recent vintage. For reasons that aren't entirely clear, heart attacks were exceedingly rare in the nineteenth century, and it wasn't until 1910 that one was diagnosed in a *living* patient. Today, by contrast, heart disease kills more than 800,000 Americans a year, and puts 600,000 more in the hospital. In 1984, the medical costs *alone* for heart disease were more than $60 billion in the United States.

But despite these grim statistics, the byword among cardiologists today is not despair but hope. There is evidence that the epidemic has peaked, and since the late 1960s the death rate from heart attacks has actually declined. This progress is due in no small part to a revolution in the drugs used to treat and prevent heart attacks, strokes, high blood pressure, and related diseases.

Physicians today know more than ever before about why these diseases occur, and what's more important, they have at their disposal whole classes of drugs that didn't even exist a few years ago. While the someday promises of mechanical hearts grab headlines, less publicized advances in drug therapy are

69

already saving hundreds of thousands of lives every year and improving the quality of life for millions more. The rate of progress is ever-quickening; beta-blockers, for example, have revolutionized the treatment of people who've survived a heart attack, and yet the first generation of these wonder drugs are already on the verge of obsolescence, supplanted by drugs having as much or more effectiveness and fewer side effects. Exciting new therapies promise to stop heart attacks even before the patient reaches the hospital, eliminate the need for expensive and hazardous coronary artery bypass surgery, dissolve dangerous embolisms, and reverse the crippling effects of strokes.

But before we review these developments, let's take a minute to look at the subject of all this interest, the circulatory system and how it works.

The subject of song and verse, the heart was believed by the ancients to be the seat of the soul and the emotions. Even today we send "heart-shaped" cards (which aren't really shaped anything like hearts) on Valentine's Day and refer to broken-hearted lovers, but modern science tells us that hearts are about as romantic as your car's oil pump. In fact, the heart *is* a pump—a lumpy mass of muscle about the size of your fist that forces blood first through the lungs to pick up oxygen and then through the body to deliver that oxygen to the body's cells. That's a more mundane job than housing the soul, but an important one nonetheless.

(Incidentally, the ancients weren't entirely off the mark when they assumed a link between emotions and the heart. It *is*, for instance, possible to die of a broken heart; the stress that accompanies the loss of a loved one has on more than one occasion triggered a fatal heart attack. Researchers have found that other emotions, such as guilt, also can affect the heart. For example, one study showed that heart attacks during sexual intercourse were more likely to occur while men were cheating on their wives than when they were faithful.)

The rest of your circulatory system isn't much more difficult to understand than the heart. The arteries and veins are essentially tubing carrying the blood to where it's needed around the body. But on closer inspection they turn out to be more than simple hoses. Veins, for instance, have a series of valves that prevent blood from flowing backward as it moves back toward the heart. Arteries are really a combination of tubing and pump. The walls of the arteries are made up of layers of muscle, which expand with every heartbeat and then contract again between heartbeats, giving the circulation an added boost.

The *coronary arteries* supply blood directly to the muscular tissue that makes up the heart. Like every other part of the body, the heart needs oxygen, and the coronary arteries' sole purpose is to supply it with oxygen-rich blood. They branch off from the aorta (the main artery that emerges from the heart) and snake along the surface of the heart itself.

Why Heart Disease Occurs

What happens when someone suffers a heart attack? What causes hypertension (high blood pressure) or angina? And why are the new wonder drugs effective against these and similar conditions?

A heart attack occurs when, for one reason or another, the heart can't perform its job adequately. As we saw, the heart is a remarkably effective muscle. Consider that if your heart beats 80 times a minute, in a single year it will squeeze blood through itself approximately 42 million times.

Every squeeze will have about as much force as you'd exert by clenching your fist. To get an idea of how hard your heart works, try clenching your fist once every second and see how long you can keep it up. You'll quickly find that your hand and arm soon begin to ache. That ache signals that the muscles are overworked, and, most immediately, that they're using up more oxygen than your circulatory system can deliver. When you consider that your heart keeps up that pace day in and day out, year after year, not only while you exercise but while you eat and sleep, you'll understand why it's so vitally important to keep that supply of fresh oxygenated blood coming to the heart tissue through the coronary arteries.

Though a heart can fail for many reasons, in most cases it's because it's not getting the oxygen-rich blood it needs. The coronary arteries themselves are the weak link in the system; they're narrow and twisting to begin with and, for a variety of reasons, tend to become blocked. When the supply of blood—and with it oxygen—is cut off, you feel pain, just as you did in your hand and arm. When you feel it in your heart, it's known as angina.

When your arm got sore from squeezing your fist, you probably stopped and gave it a rest. Unfortunately, your heart

71

can't simply stop without killing you. So to try to rest, it starts beating more slowly and with less force, which results in less blood being circulated to the body. This causes some of the symptoms of a heart attack: clammy skin, pallor, and profuse perspiration. Along with the pain from the heart attack, there is general weakness as blood flow to the brain decreases and the person suffering the heart attack feels dizzy and possibly loses consciousness.

If the blockage is severe enough, the heart finally stops beating altogether, and within a few minutes death occurs.

Hypertension

Hypertension (high blood pressure) is a disease not of the heart but of the arteries. Normally the arteries are rather springy; in addition to expanding and contracting in rhythm to the heart, they adjust themselves to the volume of the blood and to conditions within the body, stretching or tightening up as necessary to raise, lower, or maintain blood pressure. Various factors—stress, for instance, as well as diet, heredity, life-style, and aging—have a detrimental effect on the arteries. They become less springy and thus less able to adjust to changes in the body—a condition known as *arteriosclerosis* or hardening of the arteries.

Arteries are also prone to another similar-sounding condition with a similar name: *atherosclerosis*. Atherosclerotic arteries tend to become coated with *arterial plaque*, fatty deposits, that clog them, just as deposits in your house's pipes can cause your sink to back up. Atherosclerosis is responsible for clogging of coronary arteries, too, and it can cause strokes if it blocks arteries that supply blood to the brain.

These two factors—arteriosclerosis and atherosclerosis—singly or together tend to raise the pressure of the blood flowing through the arteries. That, in turn, makes the heart work harder, creating wear and tear on it, and leading to or aggravating heart disease.

This brief description doesn't begin to catalog all the possible problems that can plague the cardiovascular system, but it does provide an overview of the most common and deadly ones. In the sections that follow we're going to take a closer look at the wonder drugs that researchers have developed—and are still developing—to help heart patients stay healthy and active.

The Beta-Blockers

Fifty years ago, if you'd had a heart attack, there wasn't much your doctor could have prescribed other than bed rest, oxygen, and sedation. In many cases there wasn't even any point in admitting patients to the hospital, since there were few therapeutic alternatives beyond these basic steps. By and large doctors simply waited and hoped for the best.

But beginning in the late 1950s, doctors began to make great strides in the fight against heart disease. In 1959, Swedish doctors implanted the first pacemaker in a 43-year-old man. In 1961, researchers at Johns Hopkins University found that a combination of simple and easily learned techniques could keep heart-attack victims alive long enough to get them to a hospital and more sophisticated care. Cardiopulmonary resuscitation—or CPR as it's usually called today—has since saved countless lives and is taught in high schools, community centers, and company cafeterias. It's also taught to hospital employees and has become a mainstay of "code blue" techniques that bring hospitalized patients back from the threshold of death.

After these initial successes, medicine geared up for an all-out war on heart disease. Physicians began to realize that for hospitalized patients who had suffered a heart attack or who were at risk for one, the two things that made the most difference in their survival were intense observation and immediate therapy within minutes, or even seconds, of the onset of a heart attack. Thus were born the first coronary care units, staffed with highly trained nurses who could perform procedures that only doctors had done before.

Progress was slower on the pharmaceutical front, though. Many new drugs were developed and tested, but the first real breakthrough did not come until the discovery, over a period of several years, of the surprising versatility of a group of drugs called beta-blockers.

Propranolol (Inderal®) is the granddaddy of the beta-blocker family, and the first to be approved by the FDA for use in the United States. At the time, no one knew of the starring role that propranolol would someday come to play in the treat-

73

ment of heart disease, and few suspected that within 15 years it would be the most-prescribed drug in America.

In 1967, its sole approved use at the time was for treatment of irregular heartbeats (arrhythmias). In 1973, the FDA expanded the approved uses of the drug to include treatment of angina. In 1976, the FDA approved it for the treatment of high blood pressure, and in 1979 for migraine headaches.

All of this would have qualified propranolol as one of the most versatile drugs ever discovered, but its most important use was yet to come. It turned out to be the solution for a problem that had continued to plague cardiologists despite the many advances in treatment of heart disease.

The big problem with all these advances—the reliable defibrillators, "code blue" teams, critical care units, and all the rest—was that the patient left them behind the minute he went out the hospital door. On the one hand, doctors knew that people who'd had one heart attack were at increased risk for a second, which could strike at any time, anywhere, far from the help that had been only minutes away while they were in the hospital. And yet doctors couldn't very well keep all their patients in the hospital, waiting for a heart attack that might never come.

But in 1981 cardiologists conducting a study of propranolol found that it helped prevent second heart attacks, and that it reduced mortality rates among heart patients by 26 percent. They were so excited by this discovery that they ended the study nine months early, believing it would be unethical to withhold the drug from the control group of patients. The study's sponsor, the National Heart, Blood, and Lung Institute, estimated that widespread use of the drug could save at least 6500 lives a year in the United States alone.

How do propranolol and the other beta-blockers work such wonders? To answer that, we must begin with a look at the role that adrenaline plays in the human body.

Why Bad Days Can Be Very, Very Bad

Let's start with an example. Imagine that you've been asked to give an important speech at the next Kiwanis Club meeting. For a week you put off writing the speech, and by the day of the big event you're so worked up that you can't eat much and your throat is dry. Finally, with only twenty minutes to spare, you finish the speech and head for the meeting, but halfway there you get a flat tire.

After much huffing and puffing (and thoughts of changing your speech topic to "Road Hazards and What Should Be Done About Them"), you've got the tire changed and have stepped into a convenience store to wipe off your hands—when suddenly from outside you hear the unmistakable sound of another car rear-ending yours.

By now your heart is pounding, your knees are shaking, and you feel angry enough to yank the door off the other guy's car. After you've calmed down, you exchange insurance information, go back inside to call the police and the Kiwanis, and wait for the police to arrive. When the police car finally arrives, an officer steps out, surveys the damage, and starts writing *you* a ticket for obstructing traffic. Then, just for good measure, he notices your registration is expired and writes you a ticket for *that*.

Now wait: Let's review the sensations your body's experienced in the past two hours. First there was your dry mouth and queasy stomach, and then your pounding heart and shaky knees. And now, standing beside your wrecked and unregistered car, can't you just feel the sweat on your forehead and the blood throbbing behind your eyes? All of those sensations are caused by adrenaline. Tonight it's not doing you much good, but from an evolutionary standpoint, it's serving a very useful purpose.

Your distant ancestors didn't have flat tires and tight schedules to contend with, but they had their own problems. One of the biggest was how to avoid getting eaten by things that were bigger and faster than they were. To help them with that particular problem, nature endowed them (and, through genetics, us) with a *fight-or-flight response*. In other words, we all have a built-in overdrive system that kicks in when we're threatened by a tiger or policeman or deadline or crowd of Kiwanis.

The fight-or-flight response is governed by a complex series of interactions between your mind and body. When your brain perceives a threat, it automatically tells your adrenal glands—small organs that sit atop your kidneys—to start pumping out adrenaline. The adrenaline, in turn, quickly travels through your bloodstream to all parts of your body, acting as a sort of chemical Paul Revere to warn them that they may soon be called upon to do their best. Your digestive system shuts down and blood is diverted to the brain, helping you think quicker (and cutting down on blood loss if we're wounded in the belly). Your muscles are primed to work at peak efficiency—hence the muscular tension that results in shaky knees and twitching muscles—and your breathing becomes faster, bringing more oxygen to the blood. All of this activity is geared to help you either fight or run away. If you decide to fight, the response helps you move and think quickly—to literally stay on your toes. If you decide to run, adrenaline gives you added speed and endurance.

Unfortunately, in the concrete jungle the rules are different than they were in the good old days of tigers and other clearly defined threats. It wouldn't help you at all to get into a fistfight with that other driver and no matter how fast you run, you know the Department of Motor Vehicles will catch you sooner or later. So we've all learned that most of the time the best survival tactic is simply to stand there and act calm.

That would be fine, except nobody bothers to tell your adrenal glands. They go right on pumping out adrenaline, waiting for the big moment that never comes. While you're standing there waiting for the officer to finish writing out your ticket and trying to control your temper, your body is primed and ready to spring into action. And as you force yourself to smile at him and say, "Have a nice day," you can feel all that energy turned in on yourself. The effect on your body is something like driving your car with the parking brake on—and researchers believe that this kind of unrelieved stress is a big factor contributing to heart disease.

Now let's look *specifically* at what happens to your heart and cardiovascular system when all that adrenaline hits it, and we'll begin to see why beta-blockers are so important.

When you're under stress, the most obvious response is that your heart starts pounding much harder and faster than usual. That tells you it's working a lot harder, which in turn means it's going to need more oxygen. At the same time, the adrenaline is causing your arteries to squeeze tighter. There are two results. First, your heart has to work that much harder to pump blood through the narrowed arteries, and second, the coronary arteries can't deliver as much oxygen-enriched blood to the heart as usual.

In the normal, healthy person, these effects aren't dangerous, but if the heart is diseased or damaged, they can be disastrous. If the coronary arteries on a diseased heart tighten up, you'll feel pain (angina) which tells you that your heart is starved for oxygen. If they tighten more, or if the heart has to work harder, the oxygen shortage becomes even more severe. The heart falters—parts of it may even die from lack of oxygen—and you experience a heart attack.

This is where beta-blockers come in; researchers believe they work by short-circuiting the fight-or-flight response. The "beta" that they block are "beta receptors"—chemical codes that adrenaline must "decode" before it can act on the body's cells. If the beta-blockers get there before the adrenaline, scientists theorize, they bind with the receptors so that adrenaline can't decode them. You might say that beta-blockers are almost a "vaccine" against stress and, more specifically, against the effects of adrenaline.

The Problem with Beta-Blockers

This is not to say that these wonder drugs don't have some troublesome side effects. While they prevent your heart and cardiovascular system from "hearing" the alarm bells triggered by your adrenal glands, propranolol and other beta-blockers also prevent your other body cells from hearing the alarm too. In fact, for some patients, beta-blockers muffle the body's natural alarm system *too* much, and thereby cause unpleasant psychological side effects. Some patients report feelings of depression, fatigue, and/or lightheadedness. Patients may also experience sexual side effects, such as decreased libido or impotence.

They also tend to slow your heart rate, which can cause unpleasant and even dangerous symptoms if cardiac output or blood pressure fall too low. In addition, they can be particularly hard on your stomach, causing diarrhea, nausea, and stomach pain.

Finally, beta-blockers may cause problems for people with certain conditions or for those taking certain other types of medication. In patients with diabetes, for instance, beta-blockers may mask some of the symptoms of hypoglycemia, which means these patients must be especially attentive to their blood-sugar levels. And some beta-blockers, such as propranolol, can't be prescribed for patients who suffer from asthma or other breathing difficulties.

These side effects don't occur in all patients, and even in those who do experience them, symptoms may be relatively mild. In addition, a second generation of beta-blockers promises to reduce some of the undesirable side effects while still protecting the heart. These are the beta-1 blockers (metoprolol, for example), and they are more discriminating than propranolol and the other "nonspecific" beta-blockers. It seems not all of the body's beta receptors are created equal, and while adrenaline and propranolol affect all of them, shotgun fashion, beta-1 blockers block out the type that affect the heart while having little or no effect on the beta-receptors controlling your arteries and breathing passages. It's also possible to control, or at least reduce, side effects of beta-blockers by adjusting the dosage or by choosing from among the many variations within the beta-blocker family.

Nonetheless, for some patients side effects can't be entirely eliminated. Compared with the tremendous advantages offered by these drugs, the drawbacks may seem trivial, but not if you're the patient who's experiencing them. Fortunately, there's another type of blocker—the calcium-channel blockers—that seem to offer many of the advantages of beta-blockers without these drawbacks.

The Calcium-Channel Blockers

If your high-school class was like most, it had at least one person who turned out to be a lot more successful than anyone ever would have guessed. You know the type: some quiet kid who sat in the back of the class and never did his homework, but turns up at your 20-year reunion wearing a $400 suit and talking about his golf game and new sailboat.

In the pharmaceutical world, the calcium-channel blockers have had just that sort of unexpected success. In 1962, the first of them, verapamil, was approved by the FDA for use in the United States, but nobody paid much attention to it over the next two decades. It was just one of those thousands of little-known drugs for which nobody can seem to find much use. Its sole FDA-approved use was for the treatment of arrhythmias (irregular heartbeats), and often it wasn't even the drug of choice for that. Even if your doctor did want to give you verapamil, you'd have to be in the hospital to get it, since it was only available in injectable form and not as a pill. In fact, poor forgotten verapamil was so unpromising that nobody even thought much about how it worked or what effects it might have *other* than controlling irregular heartbeats.

All that changed, though, in the late 1970s and early 1980s. By then, cardiologists had begun to tinker with propranolol and the other beta-blockers, and their success with them prompted research into other drugs that act upon the heart. When researchers began looking around, they found that old unassuming verapamil had a lot more tricks up its sleeve than anyone had ever guessed.

The Calcium Channel

Calcium-channel blockers, as their name suggests, act on something called the calcium channel.

What is a calcium channel? That's something even your doctor would be hard put to explain to you in detail, but here's a general overview:

Your heartbeat is controlled by tiny electrical impulses; that's why doctors sometimes use electronic pacemakers to regulate hearts that don't beat the way they should. Calcium plays a key role in regulating the heart's response to this electrical signal. It flows between the heart cells and surrounding fluid through a sort of chemical revolving door—the calcium channel. The more calcium that gets through the door before the electrical signal comes, the more strongly the heart contracts and the harder it works. If a diseased heart works too hard, it might suffer damage.

Researchers have learned that one way to ease the load on a damaged heart is by controlling this flow of calcium into and out of the heart's cells. And that in turn is precisely what calcium-channel blockers like verapamil and its cousins do. They don't quite "lock" the revolving door, but they do slow it down.

This same action works on other smooth muscles (that is, the kind of muscles we can't consciously control), too. The heart is a smooth muscle; other smooth muscles line our breathing passages (and spasm like a stiff back during an asthma attack, making it difficult to breathe) and the walls of the arteries (causing high blood pressure when they tighten up). Since calcium-channel blockers work on these muscles in much the same way that they do on heart muscle, researchers are not surprisingly finding they hold promise for asthma, high blood pressure, and spasms of the esophagus. The first is particularly good news for asthmatics with heart trouble, since beta-blockers can make asthma worse.

Equally important is what calcium-channel blockers *don't* do. You'll recall that one of the problems with beta-blockers is the psychological side effects. Enter the calcium-channel blockers. In many cases they seem to offer all the life-saving benefits of beta-blockers without making you feel life isn't worth living.

If you suffer from angina, you'll be interested to learn that the calcium-channel blockers have turned out to be one of the most effective antianginal medications ever discovered. As you saw, they help your heart work less hard; at the same time they relax the coronary arteries and thus improve the supply of oxygen-enriched blood to the heart itself. The result is almost as if the drug told your heart to sit back, relax, and take a few deep breaths.

But What About Side Effects?

Of course, like all drugs, calcium-channel blockers do cause side effects in some people. Like beta-blockers, they sometimes do their job *too* well; instead of telling your heart to relax, they tell it to take a vacation. The same goes for the arteries, and so if your doctor prescribes a calcium-channel blocker he'll want to check up on you to make sure your heart doesn't start beating too slowly or your blood pressure doesn't drop too low.

Calcium-channel blockers may interact with other medications, such as beta-blockers, quinidine, methyldopa (Aldomet®), digoxin, and disopyramide. On the positive side, using nitroglycerin with calcium-channel blockers is fine; in fact, there may be some beneficial interactions.

Calcium-channel blockers aren't suitable for all patients. In particular, they're contraindicated if you have certain types of heart problems, or if you have extremely low blood pressure. And, as is true of many drugs, researchers haven't clearly established the effects on pregnant women and nursing mothers, so they recommend that pregnant women use them only if clearly necessary, and urge nursing mothers to discontinue breast-feeding if they need to take the drugs.

Calcium-Channel Blockers and the Future

What about the future of this new class of wonder drugs? Researchers are still exploring their potential, and some promising possibilities include the prevention of heart attacks and atherosclerosis, migraine headaches, Raynaud's phenomenon (a condition in which arteries in the extremities spasm uncontrollably), menstrual cramps, and premature labor. Researchers also speculate that calcium-channel blockers may someday help in the treatment of strokes, spinal-cord injuries, certain types of kidney failure, and even cancer.

That's quite a success story for the quiet wallflower from the class of '62.

Wonder Drugs That Weren't: MER/29

One of the most sordid stories of modern medicine involved triparanol (MER/29), a drug developed by the Cincinnati pharmaceutical firm of William S. Merrell. Cholesterol had been incriminated as a cause of heart disease, and it was widely believed (though never proven) that lowering the blood's cholesterol could help prevent heart attacks, strokes, and related diseases. Animal studies with MER/29 showed that it did lower cholesterol levels in the blood, liver, and other tissues. Limited clinical studies showed that it had the same effect in man, and that heart patients seemed to feel better after taking the drugs. (These studies, however, were not particularly rigorous, and the only controlled study showed no improvement in patients taking the drug.)

A 1959 symposium, sponsored by Merrell and held at Princeton, New Jersey, garnered favorable publicity for the drug in the medical community, and not long afterward, the FDA approved it for use. Hundreds of thousands of patients received MER/29, many of them simply because of high cholesterol levels in their blood.

Meanwhile, Merrell had begun receiving reports of serious side effects, including blindness caused by cataracts. Other side effects included damage to the skin, blood, and reproductive organs. In December 1960—seven months after the FDA had approved the drug—Merrell sent a warning to physicians about these problems. On April 12, 1962, the firm withdrew MER/29 from the market.

81

But later investigations revealed that Merrell had known about problems with MER/29 before the drug was approved. During early clinical testing, a laboratory technician had noted that one of the monkeys used for animal tests had apparently been blinded. She duly reported this finding to her supervisors, who decided to drop the sick monkey from the experiment, replace him with a healthy one, and falsify the experimental records to eliminate any evidence of the development of cataracts.

The laboratory technician, Mrs. Beulah Jordan, refused to sign the falsified reports, and soon thereafter quit her job. Years later, when Merrell reported that "recent discoveries" had revealed the danger of cataract formation, Mrs. Jordan told her husband the story of the cover-up. He, in turn, told the story to the members of his car pool, which, as it happened, included one Thomas Rice, an inspector for the FDA.

Rice followed up on the story, and learned that the entire MER/29 research program was riddled with lies and fraud. He learned that Merrell had indeed known of the danger of cataracts before the drug had been approved by the FDA; the firm had also known that relatively low doses of the drug could cause sterility and tissue damage in laboratory animals. But it had never passed this information on to the FDA.

After the drug was approved, Merrell invited other pharmaceutical firms to study MER/29. One of them, Merck, informed Merrell that the drug caused eye damage in rats and dogs. Scientists at Upjohn provided similar results to Merrell. By then, 300,000 patients had received the drug, and still Merrell said nothing to the FDA.

Investigations also revealed that there was more than met the eye regarding Merrell's relationship with supposedly independent investigators. An examination of the company's correspondence, for example, showed that a Merrell official had recommended providing a grant to a Los Angeles physician "rather than take a chance on his reporting negatively." A memo spoke of a paper accepted by the *American Journal of Cardiology,* purportedly by a New Jersey physician but "prepared for the most part by us." Another memo recommended payment of a personal consultation fee to a physician to avoid the possibility of alienating the doctor. Physicians at the Cleveland Clinic had written a paper describing MER/29's toxic effects; Merrell representatives had "prevailed upon" the doctors to withhold their findings for more than two years.

In 1969, Merrell was found guilty of federal criminal violations and fined a total of $80,000. Three company officials were also found guilty, receiving suspended sentences of six months each. Approximately 1,500 lawsuits were also filed against the company, with awards against the company totaling approximately $50 million.

Surprisingly, the publicity, convictions, and lawsuits all seemed to have little effect on Merrell's profits. The company's net worth, which stood at approximately $75 million when MER/29 was withdrawn from the market in 1962, had more than doubled ten years later.

The Old Standbys

In the pharmaceutical world, as in other areas of human endeavor, some of the most important work is done by "senior citizens." With all the excitement over new classes of cardiovascular drugs, you might be wondering what's become of such tried-and-true drugs as nitroglycerin. Well, it's as popular as ever with heart doctors and so is digitalis, another heart drug with an even longer history. The fact that these drugs have been around so long in no way detracts from their usefulness; rather, it's a testament to their value.

From Garden to Pharmacy:
The Discovery of Digitalis

Let's look at digitalis, for instance, a drug that was first discovered more than 200 years ago.

In 1775, Dr. William Withering was traveling through the countryside of England. Stopping at a country inn for the night, he was asked to examine a man suffering from a severe case of dropsy.

Dr. Withering had seen dropsy before, for it was a common condition of the time. Today it goes by the name of congestive heart failure, and it occurs when an overworked heart can't meet the body's circulatory needs.

The most noticeable symptom is swelling—or edema, as doctors call it—brought about because the kidneys can't eliminate salt from the bloodstream efficiently enough. As salt concentrations build up, the body responds by increasing the amount of water in the blood and other body tissues, which causes the swelling and puffiness, particularly in the ankles and feet.

Unfortunately, Dr. Withering had only bad news for his

patient. There was nothing he could do, he explained regretfully; medicine had no cure for dropsy.

On his return trip, Dr. Withering found himself stopping at the same inn. The patient was there too and, to the doctor's astonishment, he was up and about, the swelling gone.

The man told him he'd been treated by a local herbal folk remedy, the recipe of which was kept by an old woman living nearby who had a reputation of being able to cure people after doctors had given up on them. Dr. Withering, amazed by what he'd seen, tracked down the concoction, which turned out to contain more than 20 ingredients. The medicinal properties of herbs had long fascinated the doctor, and he soon found that the one effective ingredient in the mysterious potion was not some rare and exotic plant, but foxglove, a common flower in English gardens.

Following this discovery, Withering began treating dropsy with a simple tea brewed from the leaves of the foxglove plant, and found it to be effective indeed for many of his patients. After 10 years of study, he wrote a book revealing his findings.

Now you might assume that once the drug, which came to be called digitalis after the scientific name of the foxglove plant, was discovered, it only remained for others to refine its uses. Not so; though digitalis was recognized as a powerful new drug, another century and a half would pass before its true value in the treatment of heart disease would be established.

The problem was that while it was obvious *what* digitalis did—thanks in large part to Withering's meticulous observations—it wasn't clear exactly *how* it worked. Withering had noted that the drug increased the flow of urine, caused nausea and vomiting, created vision disorders, and slowed the pulse. Also, in a statement whose significance was overlooked at the time, he wrote that digitalis "has a power over the motions of the heart to a degree yet unobserved in any other medicine." Other doctors, learning of what may well have been the first miracle drug of modern times, tended to be overenthusiastic, using it for all types of swelling, no matter what the cause, and even for totally unrelated conditions. Because of this indiscriminate use, results were often disappointing, and doctors began to lose faith in the drug's effectiveness. Indeed, many stopped using it altogether.

Subsequent research only muddied the waters further. Withering had guessed that the drug acted directly on the kidneys, a notion we now know to be false, and it was not until the mid-1800s that it became clear that digitalis's effects were caused by its action on the heart.

Nearly another century would pass before doctors truly began to understand how the drug worked. Researchers in the 1930s, working with animals and with heart tissue, learned that digitalis affected the heart muscles, invigorating them and causing them to pump with more force. By beating more powerfully, the heart doesn't have to beat as quickly; this explains Withering's finding that digitalis slows the heartbeat. It also explains the drug's other effects—by strengthening the heartbeat, it almost magically reverses the symptoms of congestive heart failure. Blood passes through the kidneys more quickly, enabling them to eliminate the excess fluid and salt; a heart that has enlarged because of the added load of congestive heart failure may shrink back toward its normal size, and circulation throughout the body improves.

Nonetheless, there are limits to what digitalis can do. Sometimes heart failure is so severe that even digitalis can't help. And the drug is toxic—more so in some people than in others—and doses that are too high can cause nausea, vomiting, irregular heartbeats, even, paradoxically, worsening of congestive heart failure. Also, it has no effect on blocked coronary arteries; thus, while doctors may prescribe it after a heart attack (since the damaged heart is prone to congestive heart failure), it doesn't treat the heart attack per se, the way some of the newer cardiac drugs do.

But digitalis continues to be an extremely useful drug, and it doesn't look as though it's going to be fading from the scene anytime soon. In fact, if she were around today, there's a good chance that the old folk healer from Shropshire would be pleased—and, perhaps, a little amused—at the enthusiasm with which modern medicine has employed her homegrown remedy.

Quinidine: Another Old Friend

There are some amazing parallels between the stories of digitalis and quinidine, another important cardiac drug. Again, there was a suffering patient, a doctor who couldn't help him, and a miraculous cure. This time the setting was Vienna, just before the First World War.

In 1912, a patient appeared at the office of Viennese physician Karl Wenkebach, complaining of an abnormal heartbeat.

Like Dr. Withering, Dr. Wenkebach could offer no cure. But, the man insisted, a cure *was* possible—and he himself could provide it. Wenkebach protested; the man insisted. He would, he said, return the next morning with a regular heart rhythm. True to his word, he was back the next morning, and his heartbeat was normal, thanks to quinine, a drug already in wide use for the treatment of malaria.

We can only wonder why this patient bothered to seek a doctor when he already possessed a cure. Perhaps he was looking for a better one; perhaps he was having some fun with the good doctor. Whatever his motivation, however, modern pharmacology owes a debt of gratitude to that anonymous patient and his unknown reasons—and to the humility of such doctors as Wenkebach and Withering, who were prepared to admit that patients sometimes really *do* know things their doctors don't.

That was how the first of the "antiarrhythmic" drugs—drugs that help restore a heart to its normal heartbeat—was discovered. Or, to be more accurate, that's how the drug was rediscovered, for in 1749 a little-noted report by French physician Jean-Baptiste de Sénac cited the use of the powdered bark of the cinchona tree—from which quinine is derived—to cure "rebellious palpitation" of the heart. Today doctors prefer to use quinidine—a close relative of quinine—rather than quinine itself for treatment of irregular heartbeats because smaller doses are effective and have fewer side effects.

Nitroglycerin: Help from the Test Tube

Nitroglycerin and related drugs trace their ancestry not to some flower or tropical tree, but to the chemist's test tube. Amyl nitrite, first synthesized in 1844, was quickly found to cause flushing of the face due to the relaxation of the tiny blood vessels known as capillaries. Twenty-three years later, a young Scottish medical student by the name of Thomas Lauder Brunton suspected that amyl nitrite might also be effective against angina by increasing blood flow to the heart. He was right, as he found when he tried the drug on some of his patients. It wasn't long before nitroglycerin, which is chemically similar to amyl nitrite, was discovered to have the same effect. Both drugs are still used for treatment of angina, but nitroglycerin is by far the most common, because it is more easily administered and also has fewer side effects.

Compared with other heart drugs, nitroglycerin isn't subtle in the way it goes about its business. It simply relaxes the smooth muscles that make up your heart and arteries, with predictably straightforward results. Your heart isn't inclined to work as hard, so it needs less oxygen. At the same time, your arteries relax, so that the heart doesn't *need* to work as hard.

Nitroglycerin has the advantage of being a fairly safe drug; it's not particularly toxic to the kidneys or other systems, and it's quickly broken down and excreted by the body. There are side effects that limit its usefulness in some patients. By lowering blood pressure, it can temporarily reduce blood flow to the brain, causing dizziness. For similar reasons, it can cause feelings of weakness. And it *can,* paradoxically, cause tachycardia (a too-fast heartbeat). But these effects can be minimized by adjusting the dose.

Although nitroglycerin itself hasn't changed over the years, the ways of getting it to where it's needed have. In recent years researchers have developed several new methods that promise to make this tried-and-true wonder drug usable in even more patients.

One new way of delivering nitroglycerin (as well as some other drugs) is by means of a *transdermal patch.* For years doctors have known that nitroglycerin is easily absorbed into the bloodstream through the skin. There are nitroglycerin ointments that can be spread on the skin, and capsules that are held under the tongue or in the cheek until they dissolve. The advantage of transdermal patches, which look like big adhesive bandages, is that they regulate the delivery of the drug and so provide a constant amount of it for as long as 24 hours at a time. Their once-a-day application makes them more convenient (and thus less likely to be used improperly), while their slow, steady release of the drug ensures constant blood levels rather than the ups and downs that accompany other methods of administration. And because they make lower dosages possible, the patches help patients avoid the sometimes severe side effects that can accompany oral or intravenous administration of nitroglycerin.

There are even newer ways of using nitroglycerin on the horizon. Researchers at the University of Florida, for instance, used a cardiac catheter to inject the drug directly into the coronary arteries. Within 30 to 45 seconds, the patients' angina had disappeared.

The use of cardiac catheters to bring heart drugs directly

to the coronary arteries is a development that's on the cutting edge of modern heart therapy—and one we'll take a closer look at in the next section. It's a complicated procedure, and so the University of Florida research isn't of much practical application yet, since people with angina can't be expected to run to the nearest cardiac catheterization laboratory every time they feel an attack coming on. But it suggests that if practical means are ever developed for routinely delivering heart drugs with pinpoint accuracy, doctors someday may be able to sidestep the side effects that limit their usefulness today. And it suggests a bright future for nitroglycerin, digitalis, and quinidine. One thing, at least, is sure. As the revolution in the treatment of heart disease continues to unfold, these three drugs will not be left standing on the sidelines.

Drugs to Treat Hypertension

Hypertension is America's number-one chronic illness. More than 40 million Americans—one in six—suffer from high blood pressure. Many don't even know it, for you can have the disease for years and years before you notice any symptoms.

But just because it's invisible doesn't mean that high blood pressure is harmless. Nothing, in fact, could be further from the truth. Left untreated, hypertension can lead to strokes, heart attacks, kidney damage, congestive heart failure, and death. It's a factor in approximately 250,000 deaths every year in the United States—and more than *100 million* annual deaths worldwide. Life insurance actuaries tell us that, left untreated, mild to moderate hypertension will reduce the life span of a typical 35-year-old person by 16 years. Even the mildest form of hypertension—"borderline" hypertension—is associated with a two-to-four-year reduction in life span.

Earlier in this chapter we saw some of the ways high blood pressure can develop. Arteries can become less flexible or clogged by plaque. Continuous stress can trigger biochemical changes within the body that raise blood pressure and keep it high. Other factors contributing to hypertension include heredity, obesity, lack of exercise, diet, cigarette smoking, sex, race, age, and personality.

If hypertension is identified early enough, when it is still in the very mildest stages, the first line of defense is to try to modify some of these risk factors. Of course, we can't do anything about our heredity, age, race, or sex, but we *can* lose

88

weight, exercise more, stop smoking, and improve our eating habits. We may even be able to alter our personality; a program at Stanford University in California is intended to teach Type-A personalities (the hard-driven, success-oriented types who start blowing their horns at you *before* the traffic light has changed) how to become easygoing Type-B personalities.

But in most cases, the mainstay of treatment is with drugs. They bring hypertension down quickly and keep it down. And although they don't cure the disease (if they're discontinued blood pressure almost always shoots back up), they do prevent the serious and even life-threatening consequences that can result if high blood pressure is left untreated.

Treatment for hypertension usually proceeds in a series of steps, starting with milder drugs and moving to more high-powered ones only as necessary. The first step is usually either a diuretic (a "water pill") to reduce the salt and fluid content of the body and the blood, or a beta-blocker. If these drugs—either singly or in combination—fail to bring hypertension under control, a vasodilator is used to relax the arteries further. Finally, if all of this isn't enough, the doctor may add a drug that acts on the nervous system, such as antiadrenergic agents or ACE (acetylcholinesterase) inhibitors.

Here's a closer look at some of these drugs.

Diuretics make it difficult for the body's cells to absorb both water and salt, which are then carried by the bloodstream to the kidneys and filtered out into the urine. Hence the most common side effect is frequent urination.

The net effect is to reduce the amount of fluid in the bloodstream, which all by itself reduces blood pressure. It's like turning down the spigot attached to a garden hose, which reduces the pressure of the water coming out the other end— not a subtle mechanism, to be sure, but it works.

Because some important chemicals may be washed out with the water and salt, a doctor may prescribe supplements (most commonly, potassium supplements) to go along with diuretics.

The most commonly prescribed diuretic is hydro-chlorothiazide, although there are perhaps a dozen others as well.

Beta-blockers were discussed in detail earlier in this chapter; they reduce hypertension by making the heart work less hard. They may also reduce blood pressure by a direct effect on the central nervous system (CNS), although it isn't clear how— or even whether—they affect the CNS.

Vasodilators work directly on the muscles that make up arterial walls, causing them to relax and thus lower blood pressure. They're closely related to the antiadrenergic agents (see below); in fact, there's some overlap between the two groups.

A number of different drugs have vasodilatory effects— alcohol, for example—but there are three whose specific effects have been found to be most useful for treatment of hypertension: hydralazine, minoxidil, and prazosin.

Antiadrenergic agents could well be called alpha-blockers; they block alpha receptors just as beta-blockers block beta receptors. But rather than blocking the *effects* of adrenaline, they block its *production* by the nerve cells. Also, unlike beta-blockers, the most potent effect of alpha-blockers is not upon the heart, but upon the arteries, causing the muscles in the arterial walls to relax.

Angiotensin antagonists, which include captopril (Capoten®) and saralasin (Sarenin®), counteract the effects of *angiotensin,* a chemical produced in the body that raises blood pressure. Normally angiotensin is produced in response to a blood pressure drop as a way of maintaining equilibrium; it acts directly on the arteries to make them tighten up. Angiotensin antagonists can bring blood pressure down quickly, but can cause kidney damage and a reduction in the number of white blood cells (leading to an increased susceptibility to infection); thus, they must be used with caution.

It's easy to underestimate the value of all these various drugs. There's nothing very magical about the way they work, and they don't, on a day-to-day level, make patients feel demonstrably better. In fact, because hypertension is so often a disease without symptoms, we're usually more aware of the drugs' side effects and inconvenience than of their life-saving properties. But in terms of the number of patients helped, and the number of years added to these patients' lives, these drugs rank among the most important of any in use today. If hypertension is, as it's sometimes called, the "silent killer," then these drugs deserve the title "silent saviors."

Hope for the Future:
Unblocking Clogged Arteries

Heart attacks usually occur because the coronary arteries become clogged, and some of the most promising new drugs work to unclog them directly. These drugs offer an alternative to coronary-artery bypass surgery, in which surgeons take lengths of veins from a patient's leg and attach them to the coronary arteries to provide a "detour" around blockages.

As late as 15 years ago, coronary-artery bypass surgery was nothing more than a promising experimental technique; today, approximately 250,000 a year are performed worldwide. The operation provides dramatic relief for many patients who have suffered from angina or heart attacks, but it is not without drawbacks. It is major open-heart surgery, with all the risks that that implies. More important, it's not truly a cure; the detours themselves become clogged in time, and the operation must be repeated. Every time bypass surgery must be repeated the chances of success go down. Also, since the dangers of surgery increase dramatically with age, eventually there comes a point where the risks of the operation outweigh the benefits that can be expected. And, of course, bypass surgery can only *prevent* a heart attack; it's no help for patients who come to the hospital in the midst of an acute heart attack.

Now, however, several drugs are being investigated which may offer the benefits of a bypass without the need to undergo an extensive—and expensive—operation. All of them work by dissolving blood clots. Blood passing through arteries filled with arterial plaque tend to clot, and these clots travel through the bloodstream until they lodge somewhere, cutting off the blood supply to tissues downstream. Depending upon where they lodge, blood clots can cause strokes, heart attacks, or life-threatening pulmonary embolisms (blockages in the lung). If these clot-dissolving drugs can be given quickly enough, they can reverse these conditions before heart muscle or brain tissue dies from lack of oxygen.

Streptokinase was the first of these drugs to be studied, and it has already begun to be used to treat heart attacks in progress. Sometimes the drug is used in combination with a promising technique known as *percutaneous transluminal coronary angioplasty* (PTCA). The theory behind this procedure is as simple as its name is long, and was developed after a quick-thinking doctor in a German cardiac catheterization laboratory tried a long shot that worked.

Cardiac catheterization labs are specially equipped laboratories that permit cardiologists to run a series of tests on heart patients to determine the extent of their disease. First a long, flexible wire is inserted in an artery in the leg (or, sometimes, the arm) and threaded backward through the patient's arteries until it reaches the heart. While watching this wire on an x-ray screen, physicians can insert it into the coronary arteries themselves. Next, a catheter, a long narrow tube, is slipped over the guide wire and threaded into place. Doctors can release special dye through the catheter to see on the x-ray screen precisely where a coronary artery is clogged.

In 1979, doctors in the German laboratory were performing just this sort of procedure when, to their horror, they saw a heart attack developing before their very eyes, as the x-ray screen showed the artery they were examining become completely blocked. Cardiologist Peter Rentrop was called in to help, and in a mixture of inspiration and desperation he poked the guide wire through the obstruction, just as one might use a plumber's snake to unclog a stopped-up drain. To everyone's surprise—including his own—the trick worked. Two minutes later the heart attack had ceased.

This discovery opened up a new direction in the treatment of heart attacks, as doctors began to realize that it was possible to stop a heart attack in progress by treating it at its source, the blocked coronary artery. Subsequent research has refined the effort somewhat, and instead of a guide wire, clot-dissolving drugs and/or *balloon catheters* are now used.

A balloon catheter is just what it sounds like—a catheter with a small balloon on the end. PTCA involves inserting one of these devices into the coronary artery and simply inflating it to enlarge the narrowed passage. At first doctors believed that the balloon squeezed the arterial plaque against the wall of the artery until it was nothing more than a thin film; now, they realize, the procedure doesn't compress the plaque so much as stretch out the arterial wall. The effect is the same: a few inflations of the balloon, and blood can again flow freely through the coronary artery.

Unlike bypass surgery, the patient is fully awake during the procedure and requires only a local anesthetic where the catheter is inserted into a leg or arm. Instead of a twelve-inch chest scar and a long convalescence, the patient can look forward to nothing more than a small scar where the catheter was inserted and several hours in the hospital for monitoring.

Does all this mean that the hundreds of thousands of bypass operations still being performed are outmoded and useless? No, researchers are still studying PTCA and the answers aren't all in yet. Experience thus far has shown that about 15 percent of vessels unblocked by PTCA will close up again within a year, and studies suggest that the procedure's long-term effectiveness will be about equal to that of bypass surgery. And PTCA isn't without risks. There's a slight chance of perforating the coronary artery with the catheter, and a chance of major bleeding where the catheter is inserted into the leg or arm. More significant is the fact that in 6 to 10 percent of all cases, PTCA will bring about a heart attack, by dislodging plaque that then blocks the coronary artery further down. In these cases, immediate bypass surgery will usually be required, so it's necessary to have a heart surgeon standing by when the procedure is performed.

A major problem with using PTCA and injection of streptokinase into the coronary arteries is that it must be done in a cardiac catheterization lab. Heart tissue that's starved for oxygen may begin to die in as little as 3 hours, and after that it does little good to unblock the coronary arteries. Few heart-attack patients will be as lucky as Dr. Rentrop's German patient; three hospitals in four don't have cardiac catheterization labs, and even where they do exist it may take an hour or more to complete preliminary preparations before treatment can actually begin. That delay may be critical for reversing the damage caused by a heart attack, especially when it comes on top of delays in bringing a heart attack victim to a hospital.

Thus, in the long run *intravenous* streptokinase may turn out to be more important than *intracoronary* administration. It isn't quite as effective this way, but in most cases intravenous treatment can be started much sooner. In fact, it's very possible that paramedics will one day carry clot-dissolving drugs in their black bags, and give heart patients a shot to start reversing a heart attack even before the ambulance reaches the hospital. High-risk patients might even carry a syringe full of such

Tissue-Plasminogen Activator (t-PA)

The latest rising star in the clot-dissolving arena, tissue-plasminogen activator (t-PA), promises to overcome many of the limitations of streptokinase therapy.

Streptokinase dissolves clots—and causes bleeding problems—by destroying certain proteins that the blood needs to clot. On the other hand, t-PA homes in on existing clots, dissolving them without affecting the blood's supply of essential clotting proteins. It dissolves clots in as little as 10 minutes—a mere fraction of the time streptokinase needs to work. And since t-PA is derived from human cells, not bacteria, it doesn't stimulate the body's natural defense system.

Tissue-plasminogen activator was discovered more than 20 years ago, but until recently doctors haven't been able to study it in much detail because it was found in only tiny amounts in blood. Recent experiments with the drug became possible thanks to an unlikely source: cancerous cells that secreted large amounts of t-PA. A Belgian physician, Dr. Desire Collen, developed a culture from these cancer cells that has provided a steady source of t-PA for studies.

Recently, t-PA has been obtained from an even more unusual source: recombinant DNA techniques. Researchers have recently spliced together genes to custom-design organisms that produce relatively large amounts of t-PA. If t-PA's promise is realized and it begins to be produced on a large scale, heart patients may someday owe their lives to this living drug factory.

drugs around the way they carry nitroglycerin tablets now, and they and their family members might be instructed on how to give themselves an injection if they feel a heart attack coming on.

There are only a few drawbacks to intravenous streptokinase, but they're important ones. First, it takes a relatively long time to dissolve clots, and a lot of heart tissue can die in the meantime. Second are such complications as internal bleeding, caused by the drug's action on the clotting factors in the blood. Also, streptokinase is derived from disease-causing streptococcal bacteria, and the body reacts to it much as it would a real strep infection; patients often experience fever and other flu-like symptoms. More important, this natural resistance means that the drug won't work in patients who've recently been infected with streptococcal infections—or in those who've recently received a previous dose of streptokinase itself.

"New" Drugs Aren't Always New: A Lesson from History

With all this recent interest in streptokinase, it's often overlooked that it's been around since 1933 and that its effectiveness against heart attacks was first reported more than 25 years ago.

As early as 1949, streptokinase was recognized as a wonder drug, though for what seems today to be the wrong reasons. Certain diseases, such as meningitis, form dense abscesses of infectious material within the body. These pockets contain the disease-causing bacteria as well as clotted blood and other dead tissue. Because antibiotics are carried by the blood, and because the blood doesn't penetrate these jelly-like masses of material, these diseases tend to be very resistant to ordinary antibiotics. Researchers experimented with streptokinase as a means of dissolving these masses of dead tissue to enable the antibiotics to reach the bacteria and destroy them. It worked, and throughout the 1950s investigators reported successes in treating abscesses and cysts that had formerly been resistant to antibiotics.

Investigation into the drug's ability to dissolve clots continued, and in 1958 a study involving 24 patients showed the same effect that would make headlines 25 years later—an improvement in the prognosis of heart-attack patients who were given the drug. But these results were ignored. In fact, despite the drug's successes, its manufacturer, Lederle Laboratories, decided to abandon further development of it for treatment of arterial blood clots, due to the difficulty of controlling the drug's side effects.

Finally, in the late 1960s, two European pharmaceutical firms succeeded in producing high-quality streptokinase preparations with minimal side effects, and it began to be used to treat thromboembolisms—painful blood clots that sometimes develop in veins and arteries and which, if they break loose and travel in the bloodstream, can lodge in the lungs, heart, or brain, often with fatal results.

About this time, studies were again undertaken to investigate streptokinase's effectiveness against heart attacks. Again the studies proved it effective, and again the studies were ignored. Another decade would pass before the full potential of this life-saving "new" drug would be realized—hopefully for good this time.

Perhaps the most important lesson of the streptokinase story—for patients and doctors alike—is that medicine is as much an art as a science, and must rely to a great extent upon intuition and guesswork.

Why did doctors seemingly ignore the early reports of streptokinase's effectiveness? There are many answers to that question, of course. In the real world, most doctors are busy treating patients and—quite rightly—are wary of jumping the gun on promising new treatments until a consensus develops as to their effectiveness and safety. And while it's easy with hindsight to point to all the evidence and wonder why it wasn't noticed, in actual practice things aren't so neat. What seems in retrospect to be a smooth progression of knowledge is actually a series of breakthroughs and setbacks, hope and disappointment, and true progress can get lost in the noise, at least for a while.

6

Miracles of the Mind: Psychiatric Drugs

What is the mind? Is it, as Freud suggests, a collection of thoughts, memories, hidden motivations, and primeval urges, a dark and mysterious kingdom ruled by the id, ego, and superego? Or is it merely a supersophisticated "biocomputer," a flesh-and-blood switchboard that may someday be reprogrammed at will by scientists who understand its chemical and electrical language?

Were the paintings of van Gogh, with their strange colors and shimmering images, the result of genius or some biochemical short circuit? And, for that matter, just what is genius, or creativity, or compassion, or a sense of humor? They are parts of us, just as surely as our hands and our eyes, and yet they appear on no anatomy charts. Do they exist, or are they as fleeting as the images on our television screens, gone with the flick of a switch?

Philosophers' questions, some would say. True enough, but physicians must address them too. Throughout the history of medicine, in fact, there have existed two competing philosophies of man's psyche, and the predominance of one or the other has had profound implications on how doctors of any particular age have viewed—and treated—mental illness.

On the one hand, there is the view, which we might call the "mystical" view, that the mind is forever beyond the domain of physical medicine. The body and mind, so the argument goes, are of a fundamentally different character, and different rules

apply to each. Physicians are ministers of the flesh, whereas
the mind and soul are the exclusive domain of philosophers and
theologians. Even Freud subscribed to this idea that the mind
and the body are essentially divorced, and though he was a
physician he did not look for physical reasons to explain his
patients' mental distress. In fact, his elaborate theories of the
unconscious, and the psychoanalytic methods they engen-
dered, have more in common with the church confessional and
the theological vision of the soul than with the scalpel and the
microscope of his medical contemporaries.

Opposing this view are what may be termed the
"somaticists," those physicians past and present who incline
toward the view that the mind—or, more precisely, the brain—
is an organ like any other, and that its structure and function
are best understood using the tools of biology and chemistry.
They are likely to see schizophrenia, for instance, as a problem
not of the ego and id, but of ions and receptors.

Throughout history the mystical view has prevailed in the
treatment of mental illness. In the Middle Ages, the Church
saw abnormal behavior not as an illness at all but as evidence of
possession by the devil or invisible evil spirits, and it sentenced
many insane persons to die at the stake for failing to "repent"
of their sinfulness. For most of our own century, these invisible
spirits had new names—hysteria, repression, the Oedipus complex, and all the other darlings of parlor psychology—but treatment still consisted of luring them out and banishing them from
the unfortunate patient's mind.

However, in recent years the pendulum has begun to swing
toward the somaticist point of view. The reason is, in a word,
drugs—drugs that work to control and sometimes even reverse
mental illness. As physicians and researchers have studied
these new medicines of the mind and how they work, they have
unlocked mysteries of the brain and begun to unravel the
strange and complex methods by which we think and learn and
feel. And for the first time, there seems to be the chance to
finally bring together the two divergent views of the mind.
Research suggests that fear, passion, hope, and disappointment—the whole range of feelings and emotions that we experience—are more than mere figments or spirits; they are actual
biochemical events. In other words, they are real.

That's good news for several reasons. First, it proves that
mental illness is caused by physical or chemical factors and not
by some inherent flaw in a person's character. It dispels, for

instance, the notion that schizophrenics are running away from reality, or that people suffering from depression are simply feeling sorry for themselves. In truth, mental illness is no more the victim's fault than is diabetes or a case of the flu. (Incidentally, this type of "victim blaming" is not unique to mental illness. In the 1800s tuberculosis—or consumption, as it was usually called—was widely believed to be associated with a particular sort of personality. Thus we have inherited the image of pale and sickly poets and artists of that day—men and women whose artistic passions "consumed" them body and soul. The discovery that tuberculosis was in fact caused by a microorganism, which showed no preference for the lungs of artists over those of ordinary folk, finally laid this myth to rest.)

Even more encouraging, however, is that these discoveries hold out real hope for the control, and even cure, of mental illness. Traditional psychoanalytic therapy, by contrast, is a lengthy process with a spotty success record at best. (There's a story about a man who went to see a psychoanalyst because he was wetting the bed. After five years of analysis, he was still wetting the bed, but as he explained to a friend, "Now I know *why* I wet the bed.") Other approaches to psychotherapy, such as the behavioral methods popularized in the writings of B. F. Skinner, have had notable but limited successes and are generally ineffective in the treatment of the most severe cases of schizophrenia, depression, and mania.

How the Brain Works

This revolution in our way of looking at mental illness is based in large part on recent research into substances called *neurotransmitters,* which play a central role in the workings of the incredibly complex tangle of nerve cells within the brain.

The brain performs more functions by far than any other organ in our bodies. For example, it processes messages from our eyes, ears, and other sensory organs; it controls breathing, digestion, and the heartbeat; it generates our higher thought processes and stores information in the memory. All of these functions and more are accomplished by complex interactions among billions of nerve cells. Information is transmitted through this vast network in two ways: electrically and chemically. Sound entering our ears, for example, is transformed into tiny electrical pulses that travel into the brain via the auditory nerve. Signals from our eyes arrive in much the same way along the optic nerve.

We don't know precisely how these signals are processed when they reach the brain, but we do know that neurotransmitters have a lot to do with it. They are *chemical* signals rather than electrical ones, and they carry certain instructions from one nerve cell to another. When they reach the receiving cell, they bind with a certain protein on its surface known as a *receptor*. The chemical structures of receptors are such that they bind only with a particular type of neurotransmitter; scientists often liken the neurotransmitter to a "key" that "unlocks" its matched receptor. The neurotransmitters and receptors are involved primarily in internal housekeeping rather than the transmission of information from outside the brain. We can think of the electrical signals as the brain's incoming mail and neurotransmitters as interoffice memos.

As we'll see in the sections that follow, neurotransmitters are believed to play a role in virtually every function within the brain—sleep, alertness, pain, pleasure, thought, emotions, anxiety, memory, impulse—all the attributes we normally associate with the mind. For these reasons, the study of neurotransmitters, which is still in the very early stages, promises to unlock the secrets that were once thought to be forever beyond the reach of medicine. On a more practical level, they help explain how many different psychoactive drugs work, and they suggest new possibilities for the treatment of mental illness.

But before we focus on these new developments, let's look at how far we've come already.

Chlorpromazine: Hope for the Hopelessly Insane

Chlorpromazine—more commonly known by its brand name, Thorazine®—may well be the most maligned miracle of the modern age. Say "Thorazine" and people conjure up an image of zombielike patients sitting around playing cards. Part of the mythology of mental illness is that schizophrenics never get better, and that Thorazine helps no one but the orderlies.

But nothing could be further from the truth. Before chlorpromazine, severe mental illness was considered virtually untreatable, and people suffering from schizophrenia and other disorders were condemned to a half life of voices and visions, restraints and padded cells. And although chlorpromazine is not a cure, it has changed that prognosis for countless people, permitting many patients to lead productive and relatively normal lives outside mental institutions.

In 1955, there were more than 559,000 patients in mental institutions. At the time, mental health professionals predicted that this army of the insane would grow to 800,000 by 1975, posing a strain on societal resources as well as a tragedy of vast proportions. But when 1975 actually arrived, the number of patients in mental institutions was only 216,000—less than half as many as 20 years before. This revolution was in large part due to chlorpromazine.

The world that these patients escaped with the help of chlorpromazine was a chamber of horrors. Here, for example, is a physician's account of what life was like in a typical American mental institution just 35 years ago:

> Catatonic patients stood day after day, rigid as statues, their legs swollen and bursting with dependent edema. Their comrades idled week after week, lying on hard benches or the floor, aware only of their delusions and hallucinations. Others were . . . pacing back and forth like caged animals in a zoo. Periodically, the air was pierced by the shouts of a raving maniac. Suddenly, without notice, like an erupting volcano, an anergic schizophrenic bursts into frenetic behavior, lashing out at others or striking himself with his fists, or running wildly and aimlessly about.
>
> Nurses and attendants, ever in danger, spent their time protecting patients from harming themselves or others. . . . For lack of more effective remedies, they secluded dangerously frenetic individuals behind thick doors in barred rooms stripped of all furniture and lacking toilet facilities. They restrained many others in cuffs and jackets or chained them to floors and walls. Daily they sent patients for hydrotherapy, where they were immersed for long hours in tubs, or were packed in wet sheets . . . (Ayd, F. J., Blackwell, B., eds., *Discoveries in Biological Psychiatry*. Philadelphia: J. B. Lippincott, 1970.)

Is Valium a Wonder Drug?

From a marketing point of view, yes. Throughout most of the 1970s, Valium®—or diazepam as it's known generically—was the most widely prescribed drug in America, and it's still among the top ten.

Valium tops another kind of list, too. According to the federal government, it's the most abused drug in America—more than marijuana, amphetamine, even heroin. Valium abuse results in approximately 17,000 emergency room visits a year.

It's undeniable that benzodiazepines—a class of tranquilizers that also includes such brand-name drugs as Librium®, Xanax®, Serax®, and others—are valuable drugs. They're useful for treatment of muscle spasms, seizures, insomnia, and alcohol withdrawal, but none of these conditions comes close to accounting for their widespread use. The vast majority of benzodiazepines are, rather, prescribed for *anxiety*.

Anxiety, unfortunately, is a loose term. In its most severe form, it is a psychologically crippling disorder—witness the "anxiety attacks" that can keep agoraphobics from venturing outside the house. But on the other end of the scale, "anxiety" can mean anything from unresolved marital problems to a vague sense of dissatisfaction with one's life.

It's tempting for doctors to prescribe Valium® or other benzodiazepines for all these conditions. There are several reasons why. Patients have come to expect their doctors to provide some relief for their suffering, and knowledgeable patients may even have decided before the visit that what they truly need is a tranquilizer. Also, doctors want to help their patients, and often the surest route to this end seems to be a prescription. In addition, the many pharmacological breakthroughs of the current age—everything from antibiotics to anticancer drugs—create an atmosphere in which patients and doctors alike may tend to equate "treatment" with "drugs." Another contributing factor is that benzodiazepines, if they're not abused, are relatively safe; it's said that the only way to die from too much Valium® is to get run over by a truck full of it. (Using it in combination with alcohol, however, is another story altogether.)

But in the final analysis, there's another factor that's perhaps most important of all: advertising. Valium®, in particular, has been heavily—and often inappropriately—promoted to physicians in journal advertisements, visits by pharmaceutical representatives, and by other means. This type of advertising creates an environment in which overprescription is all too easy.

According to the AMA's *Drug Evaluations,* a handbook for

physicians on drugs and their indications, "In most cases, the individual's resolution of temporary difficulties without the use of drugs encourages the future successful and rewarding fulfillment of his/her role in society. Treatment with benzodiazepines in such cases is of little or no benefit and constitutes overmedication." Or, in plain English, don't use these drugs as a substitute for solving your problems.

So how should we view Valium® and its relatives—are they wonder drugs? If you look at the criteria we established for such drugs (Chapter 2), you'll see that the benzodiazepines fulfill all of them, with one possible exception: the ratio of benefits to drawbacks. Do the circumstances in which these drugs are truly useful outweigh their potential for addiction and abuse, and their widespread misuse as a chemical cop-out for the problems of daily living?

Perhaps; perhaps not. These drugs clearly have many friends as well as critics in the medical community. Rather than risk the wrath of either camp, we'll indulge in a small cop-out of our own. We'll call them wonder drugs—but with an asterisk.

The Development of Chlorpromazine

Most drugs are discovered rather than designed, but chlorpromazine is a different story. It was concocted in the laboratories of the French pharmaceutical firm Specia, and was intended not for the mental hospital but for the operating room. It is chemically related to an antihistamine known as promethazine, which French physician Henri-Marie Laborit had found to be effective in preventing surgical shock. Promethazine had another curious quality, Laborit learned; it produced a peculiar calming effect, under which surgical patients were calm, happy, and uncomplaining.

These qualities soon made promethazine popular with surgeons, who often used it in place of barbiturates or morphine. Laborit urged Specia's Paul Charpentier to investigate promethazine and similar compounds, and in December of 1950 the chemist synthesized chlorpromazine.

Laborit began tests with the new drug, and he soon reported that chlorpromazine worked even better than promethazine. He developed a "lyptic cocktail" consisting of chlorpromazine, promethazine, and another drug, meperidine, that induced a state of artificial hibernation. In this state, patients could be packed in ice bags until their temperature dropped to 80 degrees Fahrenheit or lower, and surgeons could perform complicated operations even on poor-risk patients.

In his research, Laborit happened to note that lower doses of chlorpromazine tended to cause, in his words, "disinterest for all that goes on around him. . . ." This effect, he noted, "let us see certain indications in psychiatry." Psychiatrists at the same hospital as Laborit agreed, and they conducted an experiment with discouraging results. Using the lyptic cocktail on manic patients, they found it to be ineffective and turned their attention elsewhere.

Another of Laborit's colleagues, psychiatrist Pierre G. Deniker, tried using chlorpromazine alone. It had little effect on depressives, he found, but in schizophrenia the effects were astounding. The drug established a bridge to patients who had been considered hopeless, even to those who had never responded to electroshock and other forms of therapy.

Within a few years, chlorpromazine and other new antipsychotics turned the field of psychiatry on its head. It unlocked the minds of thousands of patients, and freed them from a hopeless existence in the "snake pits" that passed for mental hospitals and saved countless lives. Just as significant were its effects on the minds of *psychiatrists*. The effectiveness of the drug promoted—compelled, even—acceptance of the "physical" view of mental illness over the "mystical" view.

Not that there wasn't resistance to the idea; virtually all the psychiatric drugs discovered in the 1950s and later—not only chlorpromazine but the tricyclic antidepressants, MAO inhibitors, and lithium—were met with widespread skepticism or indifference at first. But they proved so overwhelmingly effective that they were soon accepted—and along with them, the premise that the mind's ills could be due to chemistry.

Why, then, with such an impressive list of accomplishments, has chlorpromazine received a bum rap in the recent years? There seem to be several reasons.

It's true that it can cause passive, even lethargic behavior, but this must be viewed against the alternative for schizophrenic patients: raving, tormented madness. Another negative aspect of the drug is that, especially in high doses or with prolonged use, it can have troubling side effects reminiscent of Parkinson's disease—uncontrollable drooling, facial twitching, trembling hands, and other symptoms. Another factor is the distorted way in which mental illness is sometimes portrayed. Schizophrenia in particular is all too often described in romanticized—or even political—terms. It's a "window into the mind" or a "sane response to an insane world." According to this view, schizophrenics are poets, or prophets, or psychological protest marchers. But against all this wishful thinking is the reality with which psychiatrists are intimately familiar: Schizophrenia is a terrible illness, subjecting its victims to a private hell with no window to the outside world.

Perhaps the most important factor contributing to this distorted view is, paradoxically, the stigma attached to mental illness, which limits popular awareness both of schizophrenia and of chlorpromazine's effectiveness. A person whose schizophrenia is controlled by drugs, after all, isn't likely to talk about it.

One recovered schizophrenic who *has* talked about his experience—in fact, he's written a book about it—is Mark Vonnegut. In *The Eden Express,* he describes his bout with the disease, and how with the help of chlorpromazine he conquered it. His account offers revealing insights into both the myths and realities of schizophrenia and into the value and drawbacks of chlorpromazine. He writes:

> Everyone has a field day explaining schizophrenia. It's your parents, your childhood, your love life, your religion, your life style, and on and on. Usually each theory will contain just enough truth to make it irritating, but the vast majority of these theories end up giving you explanations of why you are sick rather than clues about how to get well. Besides which, most theories on this level have only poetic attractiveness and scanty, if any, objective evidence backing them up.

How Chlorpromazine Works

Although Vonnegut felt that he owed his life to chlorpromazine, he had little affection for it:

> On Thorazine everything's a bore. Not a bore, exactly. Boredom implies impatience. You can read comic books and Reader's Digest forever. You can tolerate talking to jerks forever. Babble, babble, babble. The weather is dull, the flowers are dull, nothing's very impressive.

It appears that these effects, dreary though they may be, are the very ones that help bring schizophrenics back to reality.

One way of looking at schizophrenia is that it makes the world *too* impressive, *too* exciting. The world crashes in upon the schizophrenic's consciousness like an out-of-control symphony; colors shimmer and sounds reverberate; the most trivial events seem to take on cosmic significance. In an attempt at self-preservation, perhaps, the mind finally pulls back from reality altogether, drawing into itself like a snail in its shell.

Vonnegut uses a different metaphor. Schizophrenia—the Eden Express—is a train gone wild, running faster and faster, out of control. Chlorpromazine acts like a set of brakes, slowing the train to the point where the engineer can once again control it. If the brakes are applied too much, the train slows to a crawl, but if they are released prematurely, the train once again begins to gather speed.

Precisely how from a biochemical standpoint chlorpromazine puts the brakes on schizophrenia is not entirely understood, but we do know that the neurotransmitters play a central role. One neurotransmitter in particular—dopamine—seems to have a lot to do with both Parkinson's disease and schizophrenia. (Thus it's no accident that chlorpromazine, while helpful against schizophrenia, can sometimes cause Parkinson's-like symptoms.)

In patients with Parkinson's disease, there isn't enough dopamine to go around, and as a result the nerve cells that control muscular movements tend to misfire and send garbled messages to the muscles. Thus we see symptoms such as tremors, twitching, and slurred speech.

Elsewhere in the brain, dopamine appears to play an essential role in the control of thought processes. According to one theory, one of two things happens in schizophrenia: Either the transmitting cells release too much dopamine (according to the analogy we used earlier, too many "memos" are sent) or the receiving cells are too sensitive (they overreact to the "memos"). The theory is supported by evidence that chlorpromazine's antipsychotic effects go hand in hand with its ability to block dopamine receptors, but other studies have found no evidence of excessive dopamine or dopamine receptors in the brain tissue of schizophrenics. Thus, although we know that dopamine plays a role in schizophrenia, we still don't know precisely what causes the disease.

What is Schizophrenia?

It's commonly believed that schizophrenics suffer from a "split personality." But the phenomenon of the split or multiple personality is actually an entirely distinct and much less common disorder. Traditionally, schizophrenia has been a loosely defined term, with its symptoms overlapping those of organic brain syndrome, mental retardation, Huntington's disease, and other conditions. (In fact, at one time most severely psychotic patients were labeled schizophrenic, largely because the outlook was so bleak for such conditions as manic-depressive disorder.) Because all this confusion can complicate treatment decisions, the American Psychiatric Association has established the following criteria that must be met for a clinical diagnosis of schizophrenia to be established:

- At least one of the following sets of signs and symptoms:
  1. bizarre thought-related delusions (the belief, for example, that one can broadcast thoughts to others or that others can control one's thoughts)
  2. alterations in thought form (for example, hallucinations or totally disorganized behavior)
  3. grandiose, religious, or other types of delusions, or delusions of jealousy or persecution accompanied by hallucinations
  4. auditory hallucinations (for example, hearing nonexistent voices)
- Deterioration in the patient's ability to work, interact with others, or care for himself or herself
- Persistence of symptoms for at least six months
- Onset of the disease before age 45
- Lack of evidence of mental retardation, senility, or other types of mental disorders
- No history of major episodes of depression or mania before the onset of symptoms

Despite schizophrenia's biochemical origins, external events clearly have a role in triggering psychotic episodes. Stressful situations, the use of drugs (even coffee), and even seemingly trivial incidents often spark schizophrenia, although it can also occur for no apparent reason. There's also evidence that schizophrenia runs in families; a study of identical twins raised in different homes, for example, reveals that if one is schizophrenic, the chances are increased that the second one will be as well.

Drugs that Defeat Depression

Depression is the most common form of mental illness and is one of a class of disorders known as *mood disorders.* Whereas schizophrenia and other psychoses involve disrupted thought patterns, the mood disorders affect the emotions. A person suffering from depression is as rational—as "sane"—as anyone. He can carry on a conversation, add columns of figures, and distinguish illusion from reality with ease. The problem is a lack of zest, a deficiency of good feeling.

Everyone's been depressed at times, and there's nothing abnormal about such bouts. But severe depression is another matter altogether. It drags on and on, sometimes for years. Severely depressed people may lose their jobs, stay in bed for weeks on end, and contemplate or even attempt suicide. It is more than an occasional case of the blues and most definitely requires treatment.

Unlike schizophrenia, depression—especially in its transient or milder forms—can sometimes be treated without drugs.

Nonetheless, research has shown that the disorder has much in common with schizophrenia. It tends to run in families and episodes are often brought about by stressful events. Most important, it involves changes in the chemistry of the brain and can be controlled by drugs.

A Survey of the Antidepressants

The success of chlorpromazine in the treatment of schizophrenia led researchers to study the effects of related compounds. One such researcher, Swiss psychiatrist Roland Kuhn, tested a compound called imipramine, a chemical cousin of chlorpromazine, but found it ineffective against schizophrenia. Fortunately, however, he went on to study the drug's potential for treating other types of disorders. In 1957, his persistence paid off when imipramine showed remarkable effectiveness against severe depression.

Imipramine was the first of the *tricyclic antidepressants,* the most important group of drugs used to treat depression. Other tricyclics soon followed—all with about the same effectiveness and all with similar chemical structures. They're called tricyclics because of this characteristic structure, which consists of a group of atoms arranged into three interlinked rings. (Recently a *tetracyclic*—that is, four-ringed—antidepressant has been developed, as have other novel antidepressants; they work much like the tricyclics and are usually considered members of the same class of drugs.)

The second major group of antidepressant drugs trace their ancestry to a drug called *iproniazid,* which was introduced in 1951 as an antituberculosis drug. Although iproniazid was eclipsed by a more effective cousin *isoniazid* in the treatment of TB, it was used long enough for doctors to note a curious effect that it had on patients who took it: They became uncharacteristically cheery. Many researchers noted the effect, but for five years after its introduction nobody thought about the implications of this finding for clinical depression.

One reason was that orthodox psychiatric theory at the time dismissed the possibility of an antidepressant drug. Depression was a problem within the psyche, the experts said, and even if drugs produced some alleviation of the symptoms of depression, they couldn't get to its basic psychological cause.

But by 1956, these last vestiges of psychiatric mysticism were already under attack. Dr. Nathan Kline had proved the effectiveness of the drug reserpine in schizophrenia, and news of French successes with chlorpromazine had reached America. After his success with reserpine, Kline had turned his attention to depression and conceived of a "psychic energizer"—an as-yet undiscovered drug that would put a zing back into the lives of severely depressed patients. He outlined his concept in a paper given before the American Psychoanalytic Association in 1956. This ideal drug would, he said, "reduce the sleep requirements and delay the onset of fatigue. It would increase appetite and sexual desire and increase behavioral drive in general. Motor and intellectual activity would be speeded up. It would heighten responsiveness to stimuli [and] would result in a sense of joyousness and optimism."

A few weeks later, Kline was giving another lecture at a laboratory in New Jersey, and afterward a researcher explained some experiments he'd conducted with mice. First he'd given them iproniazid, creating an apparent state of euphoria, and then he'd injected them with reserpine in an attempt to bring them down. The reserpine hadn't worked, the scientist reported.

But the first part of the experiment—the part where the mice had received iproniazid—intrigued Kline. Could this drug be the "psychic energizer" he was looking for? He began to check the literature and found that researchers had often noted the drug's invigorating effect on their patients' psyches.

And yet no one had ever suggested using it to treat depression. Almost no one, that is. Dr. Evert Svenson, the assistant medical director at the pharmaceutical firm of Hoffman-LaRoche, where the drug had been developed, had suggested to his boss that iproniazid might have some use in depressed patients, but the suggestion was met with laughter. In fact, this view was so unorthodox that Svenson later found it nearly impossible to convince Hoffman-LaRoche to supply Kline with enough iproniazid to conduct clinical trials.

Kline began with 17 "depressives" at Rockland State Hospital in New York, but soon came to the conclusion that the patients were in fact misdiagnosed schizophrenics. Next he tried the drug in 9 patients from his private practice, all of whom he knew to suffer from depression. Of the nine, one didn't respond at all to the iproniazid, another responded feebly, and the remaining seven all showed impressive improvement.

Announcing his findings during testimony before a U.S. Senate subcommittee, Dr. Kline found that the psychiatric community quickly dismissed his claims. His study wasn't scientific, many claimed (with some justification, it must be said); the evidence was merely "anecdotal."

It also happened to be correct, as later studies and a vast amount of clinical experience revealed. In the first year iproniazid was on the market, approximately 400,000 patients in the United States were treated with it.

Iproniazid was the first of a group of drugs known as *monoamine oxidase inhibitors*—or MAO inhibitors for short. MAO is an *enzyme* (a chemical whose function is to break down other chemicals) that exists in various parts of the body. These drugs act to reduce the body's supply of MAO; scientists aren't sure just how this works against depression, but it seems that MAO has a role in regulating the amounts of norepinephrine, serotonin, and other neurotransmitters in the brain.

But MAO inhibitors also act on MAO elsewhere in the body, and thus it was not a total surprise to find problems cropping up. Overdoses, it was learned, could cause hallucinations, fever, and convulsions. Also reported were damage to the liver, brain, and cardiovascular system. The most perplexing problems, though, were the *hypertensive crises* that occasionally showed up in some patients—episodes during which blood pressure inexplicably shot up to dangerously high levels. Because of these problems, MAO inhibitors soon fell out of fashion among psychiatrists, and many of them, including iproniazid, were withdrawn from the market altogether.

Some careful detective work showed that the hypertensive crises were associated with the ingestion of certain types of foods—most notably, aged cheeses. Closer investigation revealed the reason. These foods contain a substance called *tyramine* that raises blood pressure. Normally, tyramine is deactivated by MAO in the liver, but the MAO inhibitors interfered with the production of MAO and so permitted the tyramine to enter the bloodstream unchanged.

This discovery permitted the rehabilitation of MAO inhibitors. The hypertensive crises could be avoided by forgoing cheeses and other tyramine-containing foods, such as beer, wine, pickled herring, chicken liver, yeast, coffee, broad-bean pods, and canned figs. In addition, it was learned that the likelihood of hypertensive crisis was greater with some MAO inhibitors than with others, and so a few MAO inhibitors became the mainstays of treatment.

Today, MAO inhibitors have regained their place as an important tool against depression, although some psychiatrists still aren't wholly in favor of them. Since MAO inhibitors and tricyclic antidepressants work by different mechanisms, one group will sometimes work where the other has proven ineffective. MAO has also been used to treat addiction to amphetamines, shell shock, depression in the elderly, and other conditions, and research has once again been undertaken to investigate new uses for these important antidepressive drugs.

How Antidepressants Work

We saw that disturbances in the system of neurotransmitters—specifically, dopamine—are responsible for the bizarre symptoms we observe with schizophrenia. Other neurotransmitters—norepinephrine and serotonin, primarily—are involved in depression. Just as dopamine serves to regulate the brain's ability to think and to control the various functions of the body, so do norepinephrine and serotonin regulate emotions. Ordinarily they keep our emotional biochemistry safely in the middle, avoiding both the heights of euphoria and the depths of depression. When the system gets out of kilter, clinical depression or mania can result.

Scientists don't know all the details of how depression occurs, but according to one theory, it happens when receptors for serotonin and norepinephrine—the "locks" into which they fit—become altered. When this happens, so the theory goes, brain cells become overly sensitive to these mood-regulating neurotransmitters and respond inappropriately. This biochemical foul-up is translated into lethargy, hopelessness, and so on—the feelings we call depression. (If this theory is correct, it may also explain mania. Whereas depression results from receptors that are *too* sensitive, mania, which in terms of behavior is the opposite of depression, occurs when the receptors aren't sensitive *enough*.) An alternative explanation for both depression and mania is that the fault lies not with the receptors but with the cells producing the neurotransmitters—that mood disorders are caused by too little or too much norepinephrine and serotonin, rather than by altered receptor sensitivity to them.

The antidepressants, these researchers believe, work by regulating this system. Scientists suspect that they gradually alter certain receptors, making them less sensitive to the effects of norepinephrine, serotonin, and related neurotransmitters. If their guesses are correct, it would also explain why antidepressants must be taken consistently over a period of weeks before they start to work.

Problems with Antidepressants

Despite their proven effectiveness, antidepressants aren't entirely without problems. One of the most significant is misuse. As we've seen, the diagnosis of depression covers a lot of ground. As used both by doctors and lay persons, the term can mean anything from a major psychiatric illness to ordinary grief over, say, the loss of a loved one, and antidepressants are useful only for some of these conditions. The need to grieve over a loss, for example, is viewed by most doctors as a positive sign and an essential part of good mental health, and attempts to blunt it, either by pills or by well-intentioned efforts on the part of friends and relatives, can lead to later psychological problems.

The various types of depression are not at all distinct, and therein lies the problem with prescribing drugs to treat them. As a general rule of thumb, the more severe the depression, the more likely it is that antidepressants will help; similarly, the more that biological changes are associated with the depression (for instance, altered hormone levels present in the blood), the more likely it is that antidepressants will work.

But to the person experiencing it, even a "mild" form of depression is unpleasant, and if chemical relief is available—or is perceived to be available—he or she is likely to want it. Thus it's not uncommon for a physician faced with fuzzy diagnostic criteria, a patient in need of help, and a drug that he knows might help, to prescribe a possibly inappropriate antidepressant.

Unfortunately, this practice entails a cost—and not simply the financial cost of useless prescriptions. The antidepressants sometimes have significant side effects—particularly, as we've seen, the MAO inhibitors. Also, inappropriate use of antidepressants may actually make treatment more difficult, by causing behavioral changes that are erroneously attributed to the underlying disorder. For example, imipramine given to persons not suffering from depression tends to cause sleepiness, lightheadedness, and fatigue. Finally, and perhaps most significantly, misuse of these drugs can result in other forms of medical therapy being delayed or ignored.

The solution to these problems is, ultimately, more research into the causes and treatment of depression. A better biochemical understanding of the disorder may lead to more precise diagnostic guidelines and even to new types of antidepressant drugs, specifically designed to combat the various forms of depression. Such research is now under way, and together with the advances already achieved, it offers persons suffering from depression a precious commodity: hope.

Lithium: The Almost-Overlooked Wonder Drug

Of all the disorders of the human mind, manic-depressive illness is perhaps the most bizarre. Its hallmark is inconsistency, with its unfortunate victims caught on a seesaw of emotions. The *manic* phase of the illness is marked by intense activity, euphoria, incoherent raving, feelings of invincibility, and sleeplessness.

And then comes the crash—profound depression, a sense of hopelessness, and thoughts of or even attempts at suicide. It's as if the manic episode has drained the victim of any capacity for good feeling at all. But it doesn't necessarily end there. The manic and depressive phases can alternate indefinitely—sometimes for life.

Until a few years ago, this emotional roller coaster often meant lifelong institutionalization and premature death. It was one of the most untreatable of all the serious psychiatric disorders, for neither antidepressants nor such antipsychotic drugs as chlorpromazine helped cool the red-hot symptoms of mania.

That is, not until lithium salts—or lithium for short. In the past decade this drug has proved a safe and effective means of treating manic episodes, and it has become a mainstay of treatment for this condition. But the path between the drug's discovery and its widespread acceptance was a long and tortuous one. In fact, lithium very nearly vanished into oblivion, even after its antimanic properties were discovered by Australian researcher John F. Cade.

In the late 1940s, Cade was conducting a series of experiments designed to detect poisonous substances that he thought might play a role in mental illness. As part of this experiment he injected the urine of mental patients into guinea pigs. But he ran into a problem; the chemicals he was interested in didn't dissolve in the guinea pigs' blood. In an attempt to make the experiment work, he injected the guinea pigs with lithium carbonate, which he hoped would help the chemicals dissolve in the guinea pigs' blood.

But after injecting the lithium, Cade noticed an unexpected effect—the pigs became lethargic. In a flash of insight, Cade correctly guessed that lithium might therefore be of some use in treating his mental patients. He was right, and in 1949 he reported his findings in the *Medical Journal of Australia.*

Unfortunately, this brief report in an obscure Australian journal was not sufficient to attract the attention of the worldwide medical community. Cade's findings went unnoticed for nearly 20 years.

It's fortunate that Cade's findings were rediscovered, for it is unlikely that anyone else would have thought to use lithium in the treatment of mental illness. Lithium salts are relatively rare and little-known chemicals that are unrelated to any other drug. In fact, scientists still don't know how lithium tames mania. But fortunately for the patients who suffer from manic-depressive disorder, they do know one thing: It works.

Wonder Drugs That Weren't: Thalidomide

In 1956, the German pharmaceutical firm of Chemie Grünenthal introduced Contergan, a sleeping pill that quickly dominated the market in West Germany—in large part because of its reputation for safety. Animal tests showed that large doses given to animals produced no ill effects, and clinical trials showed it to be safe in humans. It was available without a prescription in Germany; a special liquid form for children earned the nickname "West Germany's babysitter." It was also useful for nausea in pregnancy, an indication for which it soon gained widespread popularity.

Contergan—which would soon become infamous under its generic name, thalidomide—was soon being marketed throughout Europe, while plans were laid to launch the drug in the United States. In 1960, the William S. Merrell Company obtained the U.S. patent and applied to the Food and Drug Administration (FDA) for permission to market the drug.

Under the then-current rules, the FDA had only 60 days in which to approve or deny the application, but the FDA medical officer responsible for approving the application, Dr. Frances Kelsey, had doubts about this drug. There had been a few reported cases of nerve disorders linked to the drug, and there was scant evidence of the drug's long-term effects. In addition, her previous research led Dr. Kelsey to suspect that thalidomide might have unsuspected effects on the fetus. The doctor used the only delaying tactic she had available to her; she ruled that the application was incomplete and requested more data.

Merrell began pressuring the FDA to approve the drug, with company representatives calling and visiting repeatedly, but Dr.

Kelsey and the FDA still refused to approve the drug. A year later, Merrell was still waiting, and poised to launch an all-out information onslaught on the FDA.

Then, suddenly, the bubble burst. On November 30, 1961, Grünenthal announced that it was withdrawing Contergan from the market in West Germany. Evidence had surfaced that "West Germany's babysitter" had a terrible side effect. It sometimes caused flipperlike limb deformities in children born to women who took the drug while they were pregnant.

In all, as many as 8,000 children were born with birth defects caused by thalidomide. And despite the FDA's refusal to license the drug, the thalidomide tragedy did reach the U.S.; Merrell had distributed 2,500,000 "samples" of thalidomide tablets to U.S. physicians; at least 624 women took the drug while they were pregnant. It isn't known how many children in the United States suffered birth defects as a result, but it is known that Merrell settled at least 10 cases out of court.

The thalidomide tragedy was a pivotal event for the FDA and the U.S. pharmaceutical industry. The news broke just as Congress was considering new legislation to toughen the FDA's authority and require more extensive preclinical testing by the drug companies. The legislation hadn't been expected to pass, but after the thalidomide story emerged, its sponsors were able to marshal public support for the bill and ensure passage of what became known as the Kefauver-Harris Amendments of 1962.

The Conquest of Epilepsy

Few diseases in history have been as misunderstood as epilepsy. Three hundred years ago, epileptics were often burned at the stake, accused of witchcraft, or considered to be possessed. Later, it was considered a form of insanity or retardation.

And it was, until this century, untreatable. In the nineteenth century, its victims were often confined to "epileptic farms" or mental hospitals, and their "care" consisted of nothing more than straitjackets or other restraints.

The revolution sparked by the discovery of effective antiepileptic medications is even greater than for schizophrenia. Gone entirely are the epileptic farms; these days epilepsy is an almost invisible disease. In the vast majority of cases, these drugs are but a small step removed from a *cure,* preventing virtually all seizures when taken regularly.

Today, two classes of drugs are used most widely for epilepsy, and for the thousands of patients suffering from this disease they are indeed wonder drugs. No longer does epilepsy have the grim prognosis that it had until this century. Now it's usually possible to control epilepsy so completely that patients can live entirely normal lives and go for years without a seizure.

The first reported use of a drug to treat epilepsy appeared in a 1912 article in a German medical journal. The drug was *phenobarbital,* which traced its history to barbituric acid, a compound discovered in 1864 by German chemist Adolph von Baeyer.

Phenobarbital and the other *barbiturates* proved to be inexpensive and effective therapy for most forms of epilepsy, and their use sparked a profound revolution not only in the treatment of the disease, but in the public perception of it. This revolution was like the one that would occur half a century later with schizophrenia. The "epileptic farms" and asylums emptied, their padded cells and straitjackets no longer needed.

But although phenobarbital continues to be useful in the treatment of epilepsy, it has always had some drawbacks. The barbiturates are best known today as powerful sedatives, and though the doses required to control epilepsy are relatively low, they do cause drowsiness, fatigue, and lethargy. Thus, it wasn't long before researchers began searching for an alternative. Drs. H. H. Merritt and T. J. Putnam began testing the ability of various chemicals to suppress convulsions in laboratory animals who had been subjected to electroconvulsive shock treatment.

Their search led them to phenytoin (Dilantin®), a drug that is chemically related to the barbiturates but controls seizures without causing drowsiness or sedation. Phenytoin was good news to epileptic patients for two reasons. First, it improved their quality of life, and second, it reinforced the idea that epilepsy is not a "mental illness" in the sense that schizophrenia or depression is. That is, by proving that epilepsy could be controlled without affecting the patient's thought processes, phenytoin showed that the two had little to do with each other.

This insight has been borne out by modern electrical studies of the brain, which show seizures to be miniature electrical storms within the brain. As we've seen, the brain is always full of electrical activity. Usually it's organized and purposeful activity, a sort of biological version of telephone and cable television transmission with thousands of "channels" sending and receiving messages between the body and the brain, and between the various parts of the brain.

Just as a summer thunderstorm can disrupt your telephone service, so can unpredictable bursts of electricity within the brain bring on seizures. Usually seizures start at a certain *focus* (plural: foci)—an area that can be anywhere within the brain and that, for one reason or another, sometimes send out a burst of disorganized electricity. When this electricity reaches nearby cells, it causes them to discharge, in turn giving off more electricity.

The effect is a chain reaction that spreads throughout the brain, disrupting its finely tuned communication system. As these bursts of "static" garble messages to the body and the various parts of the brain, an observer may see the classic signs of a grand mal seizure—unconsciousness and uncontrolled spastic movements—but seizures take many different forms that are not so dramatic.

Eventually, the brain reestablishes equilibrium, and the seizure ends. Usually, however, there's a temporary residual effect, with depression and fatigue being common symptoms. These feelings may last anywhere from a few hours to a day or longer, and may be compounded with stress or worry over the seizure. Often the best thing a person can do after a seizure is to get a lot of sleep.

Despite all the research that has been done into epilepsy, nobody knows just what it is that causes cells in the foci to discharge in the first place. Sometimes there's a pretty obvious cause—a brain tumor, for example, or a blow to the head—but more often than not, the cause is a mystery. And to make the question even more complicated, it appears that sometimes there is no clearly defined focus of abnormal electrical activity at all; in such cases a seizure may begin anywhere in the brain.

Fortunately, however, the antiseizure drugs work a little farther down the line. Phenytoin appears to suppress abnormal electrical discharges of cells, while barbiturates seem to limit the sensitivity of cells to such discharges. Put another way, phenytoin controls a cell's electrical *output* while barbiturates control the *input*. Either way, the drugs effectively break the electrical chain reaction that leads to a full-blown seizure.

Other drugs have since been discovered that are useful in the treatment of epilepsy, most of them chemically related to both phenytoin and the barbiturates. The precise drug and dosage that a doctor prescribes depends on several factors—the relative effectiveness of the various drugs against different forms of epilepsy, the age of the patient, and the severity of side effects. Together these drugs offer doctors a powerful array of therapeutic tools. For patients, they offer something that has been denied epileptics throughout history: the chance for a normal life.

From Junkies to Junk Food: Drugs to Treat Addiction

Addiction is an illness of paradoxical origins. On the one hand, it can trace its lineage back to the beginnings of recorded history. Around 700 B.C., Homer recorded what in all probability is a description of opium: "Now Helen, daughter of Zeus, turned her thoughts elsewhere. Straightaway, she cast into the wine of which they drank, a drug which quenches pain and strife and brings forgetfulness to every ill." Archaeological evidence suggests that opium was even known to the pharaohs.

Opium in its unrefined state is addicting, but it's an inconvenient drug to use. Usually it was smoked or taken by mouth; occasionally it was inhaled through the nose like cocaine. But these methods made it difficult to take in large amounts of the drug, and so limited both its effects and its potential for serious abuse.

It remained for nineteenth-century science to provide the tools that would transform opiate addiction from an exotic curiosity into the major public-health problem that it is today. The first step was the synthesis of opium derivatives—morphine and heroin, primarily—that could produce pain relief and, in relatively high doses, an almost magical sense of well-being. The second was the invention of a device that could bring about these effects almost immediately—the hypodermic needle.

These developments had a dual set of consequences, one bad and one good. On the one hand, it spawned one of the gravest social ills of our time. But sometimes overlooked in the discussion of the opiates—or narcotics, as they're often called—is that they offered doctors a powerful new means of controlling pain.

Make no mistake, the narcotics are miracle drugs just as surely as penicillin or cyclosporine. They're legitimately prescribed for everything from diarrhea to the pain of terminal cancer. In fact, if you've ever been hospitalized for major surgery, chances are good that you've received morphine so pure that an addict would salivate at the thought of it.

But despite their place in medicine, the nonmedical uses of narcotics have earned them a Dillinger-like reputation among police officers, customs agents, and public health officials. It wasn't always so; a hundred years ago, opium was the Valium® of its day—a drug with a slightly naughty reputation, but still acceptable, even fashionable, among the well-to-do. It wasn't illegal—you didn't even need a prescription—and it found its way into many patent medicines, where it was sometimes combined with alcohol, cocaine, or other potent drugs. (Incidentally, one such preparation—now available by prescription only—that has survived into modern times is paregoric. A mixture of opium and other substances, it's officially listed as an antidiarrheal medication. Unofficially, it's been used by more than one mother to quiet a fussy baby.)

In the early part of the twentieth century, increasingly widespread recognition of the hazards of opiate addiction led to the passage of stringent laws in the United States governing their use. No longer the fashionable parlor drugs of Victorian days, all narcotics were, by 1919, outlawed except for medical uses.

The Complexities of Curing Addiction

But the passage of these laws failed to halt the spread of addiction. It is in fact doubtful whether any laws could curb addiction, for everything we know about it suggests that it is a disease rather than a crime.

And it has proved to be a difficult disease to treat. One reason is that it is two-pronged, having both a physical aspect and a psychological aspect. With prolonged narcotics abuse, the body becomes physically dependent on the drug, and withdrawal can be an extremely painful and dangerous process. At the same time, the mind-altering effects of narcotics can create an almost uncontrollable psychological dependence.

Though closely related, these two problems are distinct. It's possible, in fact, to be physically but not psychologically addicted to narcotics—as sometimes happens to hospitalized patients receiving morphine for severe pain. Similarly, psycho-

Endorphins and the Brain

It was research into the problem of narcotics addi laid the groundwork for our understanding of the peptide neurotransmitters and how they function within the brain. The first type of peptide neurotransmitters to be discovered were the *endorphins,* whose existence was hinted at by some of the features of opium addiction.

It's well known, for instance, that various narcotics tend to be interchangeable in many respects. Thus, someone who's addicted to heroin can satisfy his craving with morphine or other derivatives of opium. (This effect is the basis for methadone-maintenance programs. Methadone is a powerful narcotic with many of the same effects as heroin. The main difference is that it can be given by mouth as well as by injection, and therefore it's suitable for outpatient programs in which, theoretically, addicts are gradually "weaned" from heroin.) Scientists also know that all the opiates share certain basic chemical structures, and they guessed that these structures must have something to do both with their pharmacologic properties (the ability to blunt pain and induce euphoria, for example) as well as with their addictive potential. This line of reasoning suggested the existence of receptors on brain cells that were activated by opium and related drugs. Further research showed that these receptors did in fact exist.

But there was still one unanswered question: Why? Why would the human brain have receptors for a substance that naturally occurred only in the seed pods of a certain species of poppy? And why are the opiates such powerful and addictive drugs?

Perhaps, researchers surmised, the opiates mimic some substance produced within the brain. They guessed that this homegrown opiate, if it existed, would play an important role in regulating certain functions of the brain. From the narcotics' analgesic properties, for example, they surmised that it had something to do with how the brain interpreted and responded to the nerve impulses signaling pain. From their euphoric effects, they concluded that it also played a role in the perception of pleasure.

In 1973, researchers at New York University, Johns Hopkins University, and the University of Uppsala in Sweden independently identified opiate receptors in the brain. Not long afterward, tiny traces of opiatelike substances—the endorphins—were also discovered.

logical dependence often occurs in the absence of physical addiction, and in the case of street addicts, almost always precedes it.

Recent research has yielded two types of drugs—clonidine and the narcotic antagonists—that help overcome physical and psychological addiction, respectively. But this area of research involves more than the treatment of hard-core drug abuse; it also points the way toward a deeper understanding of the nature of pain and pleasure, and suggests exciting new ways of treating alcoholism, obesity, and other "addictions" of daily life.

The key to the puzzle of addiction, like so many other mysteries of the mind, is held by those intercellular messengers, the neurotransmitters (see box). When researchers began to study the role of the endorphins in the brain, they discovered that, unsavory as it sounds, we're all junkies in a sense. The endorphins—naturally produced substances that are much more powerful than the most potent narcotics—are essential to our subjective feelings of well-being.

This truth suggested a new way of looking at both the physical and psychological aspects of narcotics addictions. Narcotics, by mimicking endorphins, "fool" the brain into adjusting its chemistry in response. Narcotics, acting together with already-present endorphins, tend to overstimulate the pleasure receptors in the brain. When such drugs are used on a regular basis, the brain tries to restore equilibrium by cutting back on the amount of endorphins it produces, and by reducing the number of opiate receptors. In this way, narcotics become a necessary part of the brain's status quo, which explains the phenomenon of *tolerance,* in which chronic narcotics users need ever-larger doses just to feel normal.

Now, consider what happens when this steady source of narcotics is suddenly stopped—say when a heroin addict doesn't get his fix. It's as if the bank suddenly calls in its loans. The brain is caught short, and the fun stops. With both endorphin production and the number of opiate receptors reduced, the pain-pleasure pendulum swings back with a vengeance.

This is why the "cold turkey" approach to narcotics detoxification is so painful. Until the brain can reestablish equilibrium, it craves relief; it longs for any chemical—whether from the body or from the poppy—that can activate its stunted crop of pleasure receptors and eliminate the pain.

Until recently, anyone trying to kick a narcotics habit had but two choices—"cold turkey" or slow, gradual detoxification. The choice was like the decision you have when removing a Band-Aid®—you can rip it off quickly and have it hurt a lot for just a little while, or pull it off slowly and have it hurt a little for longer.

Both have disadvantages. The cold turkey approach, in addition to being painful, isn't always successful; once he returns to his old life, the detoxified addict often relapses into his heroin habit as quickly as he gave it up.

The gradual approach to detoxification is accomplished by the use of methadone. But methadone is an opium derivative like heroin and morphine, and it doesn't cure heroin addiction; it simply substitutes one addiction for another. It does possess a quality, however, that has some value in a gradual detoxification scheme: it can be taken orally. In a methadone program, an addict substitutes an erratic and illegal habit for a controlled and legal one. Once that is accomplished, the methadone doses are slowly decreased until eventually dependence is broken.

At least, that's the way it works in theory. But there are some pretty obvious flaws in the plan. First, detoxification takes a long time, and many participants cheat or simply drop out of the program. Also, methadone detoxification tends to run against the tide; it's an attempt to *reduce* the dosage of narcotics at the same time that tolerance effects make the body crave *increasing* doses.

These problems always made the treatment of narcotics addiction a difficult and painful process, with many setbacks and relatively few long-term successes. But events of the past few years have rendered these scenarios as obsolete as surgery without anesthesia. Clonidine now makes possible rapid and virtually painless detoxification, and naltrexone helps ensure that a once-kicked habit stays kicked.

Clonidine and Lofexidene

Clonidine began life as a medication for high blood pressure, and it's still widely used for that purpose today. It lowers blood pressure by acting on a type of receptor in the brain known as an *alpha receptor,* which in turn relaxes the muscles that make up the walls of arteries (see Chapter 5). It is clonidine's effects on alpha receptors that also make it useful in eliminating the symptoms of withdrawal.

To understand the role of the alpha receptors, we must consider the anatomy of addiction. Deep within the gray matter of the brain is a group of nerve cells called the *locus ceruleus*—the LC for short. The cells of the LC are loaded with opiate receptors, which suggests that they play a vital role in the processing of pain-and-pleasure signals.

Though they're important, the LC cells are sort of the Hell's Angels of the brain—their mission is to make people feel bad. When they're active, they send out panic signals that result in all sorts of unpleasant feelings—pain sensations, chills, excessive sweating, and so on. Normally, they're kept happy (and, thus, quiet) by steady doses of endorphins. As we saw, though, the addict suffers from an endorphin shortage, and his LC cells suffer from a shortage of opiate receptors. As long as the addict gets his fix, that's no problem; narcotics take up the slack.

But take away the external source of narcotics, and the LC cells stop smiling and start causing trouble. They tell the stomach to start cramping, the sweat glands to start sweating, and the muscles to start aching.

The trick that makes clonidine work is that the LC, in addition to its role in the regulation of pain and pleasure, is also wired into the autonomic nervous system—the same system that controls blood pressure. The LC cells have not only opiate receptors, but also alpha receptors. Thus they can be placated by clonidine even though they're not getting their usual fix of endorphins or narcotics.

The results are dramatic. Almost immediately the pain and physical symptoms of withdrawal are eliminated. If clonidine therapy is begun before detoxification begins, the addict experiences withdrawal that is entirely pain-free.

Now, keep in mind that although clonidine calms the LC cells, it does so by way of an entirely different pathway than narcotics; it's not a substitute for heroin in the sense that methadone is. This fact, as you might expect, gives it a number of important advantages over methadone. It's nonaddicting, causes no euphoria, permits narcotics to be discontinued immediately, and permits rapid detoxification (generally within two weeks).

There are, however, some drawbacks to clonidine, mainly its tendency to cause drowsiness and low blood pressure. Because these side effects are sometimes severe, clonidine detoxification should be done in a hospital. To overcome these problems, doctors have recently tried a related drug called lofexidene.

Lofexidene also lowers blood pressure, but not as severely as clonidine, and it doesn't usually cause drowsiness. However, it does bind to the same receptors as clonidine, and thus it works nearly as well in preventing withdrawal symptoms. Although lofexidene hasn't yet been studied as extensively as clonidine, this combination of features may eventually make it the drug of choice for narcotics detoxification.

Naltrexone

But the addict who is successfully detoxified is only half-way home. Staying on the wagon is difficult, especially when he or she returns to the real world and all the temptations and stresses that gave rise to the original habit. The traditional approach to preventing relapses has been through counseling and therapy, attempts to manage the stresses leading to narcotics abuse and to change behavioral patterns that perpetuate it. Sometimes this approach works; often, however, it doesn't.

Naltrexone, however, can help in a way that counseling can't. It simply removes temptation—or, rather, the ability to be tempted. By binding to opiate receptors, it entirely blocks the effects of narcotics. Someone taking naltrexone can take all the narcotics he can get his hands on, and he won't feel a thing. Doses that otherwise would literally kill him leave him unaffected.

A closely related drug, naloxone (Narcan®), possesses these same properties, and has been used since its introduction in 1971 by paramedics and emergency room physicians to reverse narcotics overdoses that previously would have been fatal. But naltrexone has two features that naloxone doesn't. It can be given by mouth, and its effects last for days rather than hours. That makes it possible to establish outpatient programs in which cheating is chemically impossible.

Of course, motivation is still the most essential factor. Recovering addicts who drop out of the program will, after a few days, be as susceptible to addiction as ever. But naltrexone gives a welcome boost to this motivational factor. No longer prey to every passing moment of weakness, the patient is faced only with the responsibility of performing a single, focused act: taking his medication. The difference is revealed in the statistics: 45 percent of patients in a naltrexone program at the Connecticut Mental Health Center in New Haven stuck with it for at least six months; according to Director Herbert Kleber, M.D., "not long ago a 20 percent retention after six months was considered good." At Fair Oaks Hospital in New Jersey, the retention rate at 6 months for physicians, executives, and other working addicts is approximately 60 percent. Within these statistics lie a revolution in the long battle between man and the poppy—and hope for solving one of the most troubling social ills of our time.

Endorphins and the Theory of Addiction

Narcotics addiction may be a social problem, but for most of us it's not a personal problem. Or is it?

To a greater or lesser degree, virtually everyone is addicted to something. More than 80 million Americans, for example, suffer from obesity. Some people are addicted to cocaine, or alcohol, or cigarettes. The subject of the addiction need not be physical; runners, for example, often report a "runner's high," and become depressed and irritable if the weather or other circumstances keep them from lacing up their sneakers and hitting the streets. Similarly, people can become addicted to power, or the feeling of falling in love, or driving fast cars.

It seems, in fact, that people have the innate capacity to become addicted to almost anything. And despite their seeming diversity, all of these addictions have remarkable similarities. Tolerance, for example, is a feature common to many addictions: to experience the same "high," the daredevil, for instance, must take bigger and bigger risks; the overweight person eats even past the point when he feels full.

The common thread to all these addictions, according to one promising theory, may lie with the endorphins in the brain. Remember that these naturally occurring narcotics are far more powerful than heroin or morphine, and seem to be responsible for producing sensations of pleasure. When you bite into a candy bar or fall in love, it feels good because endorphins are being released in your brain. An oversimplified, but useful, way of looking at this theory is that pleasure equals endorphins equals narcotics equals potential addiction.

Not surprisingly, our brains like the feelings they get from these endorphins, and they'll look for ways to keep them coming. Thus it's our craving for these natural narcotics that propels us back to the Seven-Eleven looking for more candy bars (or, perhaps, the chance to fall in love with the girl behind the counter). A certain amount of this craving is normal—in fact, it's a necessary source of motivation for everything from cooking dinner to keeping a job—but there's a fine line between the right amount and too much. That line marks the beginning of addiction.

This, in a nutshell, is what's known as the endorphin theory of addiction—that all sorts of compulsive and self-destructive behaviors are ultimately explainable by endorphins. But as appealing and elegant as the theory sounds, how can we tell whether it is in fact accurate?

Well, some interesting observations have tended to support the theory. A number of patients in the drug rehabilitation program at Fair Oaks Hospital in New Jersey, for example, lost between 5 and 11 pounds at a rate approaching two pounds a week while receiving naltrexone; all reported a much-diminished appetite. Other researchers have found similar effects when naltrexone is given to persons who have never been addicted to narcotics. These results point to a connection between obesity and narcotics addiction, and suggest that naltrexone or related drugs may one day help overweight people "detoxify" themselves from ice cream and Twinkies, just as it now helps recovering narcotics addicts.

Also supporting the endorphin theory of addiction is the fact that former heroin addicts are at high risk for alcoholism, especially when narcotics aren't available. Evidence suggests that alcohol causes the brain to produce substances that bind with the opiate receptors, and researchers have discovered that naloxone can reverse the depressant effects of alcohol, can bring persons out of an alcohol-induced coma, and can prevent such alcohol-induced symptoms as slurred speech and lack of coordination. Similarly, clonidine has proved helpful for persons trying to give up cigarettes.

All of this supports the idea of a close link between endorphins and addiction, and it suggests the potential for discovering exciting new drugs to overcome our everyday addictions. Imagine, for instance, a diet pill that has none of the dangers or unpleasant side effects of amphetamines. Imagine two-pack-a-day smokers finally kicking their habit once and for all. Imagine the lives that would be saved by eliminating just these two addictions.

And, on the lighter side, imagine how life could be improved in countless tiny ways: No more temptation at the supermarket checkout counter. No more candy wrappers stuffed furtively under the front seat of the car. No more Adidas addicts clogging our back roads and bike paths in pursuit of their "high." O brave new world!

Wonder Drugs That Weren't: Cocaine

One of the most popular all-purpose remedies of the nineteenth century was cocaine. In 1885, the pharmaceutical firm of Parke-Davis called cocaine "the most important therapeutic discovery of the age." Corsican chemist Angelo Mariani offered it in wine, elixirs, tea, and other media. One of Dr. Mariani's colleagues reported that he had used "Mariani wine" to "restore the voice of many lyric artists." Another claimed that he had used it to treat a young woman suffering from a laundry list of disorders, from headache and dizziness to night sweats and "sitting up late at night." A month of treatment and the woman's condition was "most satisfactory." Cocaine was also a popular treatment for hemorrhoids, and at one time Sigmund Freud recommended its use for treatment of morphine addiction, asthma, impotence, and a variety of other ailments.

Nearly a hundred years later, in the 1970s and '80s, cocaine again was fashionable, albeit illegal. There was widespread belief among its users, buttressed by reports in underground publications, that cocaine was a safe and nonaddicting high.

All of this, unfortunately, was just so much wishful thinking. Cocaine is, perhaps, the most addicting drug known. Experiments with monkeys show that if they are provided with an unlimited supply of cocaine, they will prefer it to other drugs, sex, or even food, and eventually they will use it until they die of an overdose. In addition, cocaine abuse has many well-documented side effects, including respiratory problems, ulceration of the delicate membranes of the nose, sleep disorders, impotence, cardiovascular problems, and long-term depression.

As for cocaine's "medicinal" properties, they are equally illusory. Although research continues into the drug's therapeutic potential, thus far it has only found use as a local anesthetic. And since the discovery of lidocaine, it hasn't even been used for that purpose. Undoubtedly, cocaine can make you feel wonderful—but it's no wonder drug.

The Future of Psychoactive Drugs

As we learn more and more about neurotransmitters, receptors, and how they work, we are gaining new insights into the function of the brain and ways of treating it when things go wrong. Just recently, for instance, research at Fair Oaks Hospital provided strong evidence of a link between cocaine abuse and dopamine—the same neurotransmitter that is the key to understanding schizophrenia and Parkinson's disease.

Evidence suggests that cocaine stimulates the brain's production of dopamine in the short run, but depletes it in the long run. When chronic cocaine abusers stop taking the drug, they report such unpleasant symptoms as depression, fatigue, disturbed sleep and appetite, and irritability—not to mention a strong desire for cocaine—and these symptoms appear to be linked to a deficiency of dopamine in the brain.

Proof of this link came from a trial of bromocriptine at Fair Oaks. Bromocriptine, a drug sometimes used in the treatment of Parkinson's disease and other disorders, is known to reverse the effects of chronic dopamine depletion. Sure enough, cocaine abusers trying to kick the habit reported that bromocriptine was invaluable in getting them over the hump.

Further proof came when one of these cocaine abusers was given thioridazine (Mellaril®) for hallucinations. Thioridazine blocks dopamine receptors and thus would be expected to intensify the unpleasant effects of cocaine withdrawal. Another direct hit; the patient reported an intensified craving for cocaine while taking thioridazine.

These successes illustrate two important facts about this exciting area of research. First, they underscore the fact that we now possess an insight into the brain never before achieved in the history of medicine. Clonidine, naltrexone, bromocriptine—all of these discoveries offer evidence that this basic research is clearly on track.

Also, these results point out the vast amount of interplay between the various brain functions. Dopamine, for example, plays a role in schizophrenia, depression, Parkinson's disease, cocaine addiction, and other disorders of the mind; other neurotransmitters also have multiple effects. This, in turn, suggests the possibility of using "old" drugs in new ways. Just as researchers have found new uses for clonidine, lofexidene, and now bromocriptine, current research hints at a possible role for narcotics in the treatment of schizophrenia and other diseases. Nobody knows yet just where all this investigation will eventually lead, but one thing is sure. By firmly establishing the biochemical basis of mental illness, doctors have made mental illness more comprehensible and less mysterious than ever before. With any luck, we have banished the ancient "demons" forever.

7

Painless Wonders:
Anesthetics and
Analgesics

Of all the bad things that can happen to our bodies, pain and death are the two we can count on. Perhaps that's why mankind has always had such a fascination with substances that can relieve pain, and why painkillers are perhaps the most ancient of all wonder drugs. We've already seen that opium was known to the ancient Greeks, but it wasn't the only pain reliever of the day. Good old-fashioned alcohol has been prized since prehistoric times for its mind-altering and painkilling properties and has been used in virtually every corner of the world. To the Greeks it was sacred, a special gift from the god Dionysus. Similarly, the Egyptians believed that Ra, the Sun God, had given mankind the mandrake root, which yielded a powerful anesthetic. The hemp plant, or marijuana, is another ancient source of pain relief, and the Greek writer Herodotus informs us that its derivative hashish was both eaten and inhaled in ancient Greece. In the New World, South American Indians have used coca leaves (from which is derived cocaine and a flavoring used in Coca-Cola) for longer than anyone can remember, both for its euphoric and anesthetic effects.

The ancients understood that painkilling drugs were not only useful in relieving suffering caused by illness or accidents, but also helped patients endure painful but necessary operations. A Greek philosopher by the name of Apuleius, who lived about 150 years after the birth of Christ, offered this advice: "If anyone is to have a member mutilated, burned or sawed let him drink half an ounce with wine, and let him sleep till the member is cut away without any pain or sensation."

The Decline of Painkillers

Unfortunately, such enlightenment was lost in the centuries following the fall of the Roman Empire, and the Middle Ages saw the development of a peculiar attitude toward these long-standing benefactors of mankind. A French document from the sixteenth century, for instance, tells of the arrest and trial of one Nicolas Bailly, a barber-surgeon, on charges that he'd practiced witchcraft by giving a narcotic to a patient before operating on him.

With narcotics forbidden, medieval surgeons had to resort to less effective means of anesthesia. One alternative was alcohol; a less pleasant one was the practice of throttling—that is, pressing on the carotid artery in the patient's neck until he passed out. Sometimes the prescription was the proverbial bullet to bite on and a few burly assistants to hold the victim/ patient steady.

As might be expected, such methods were not met with enthusiasm by patients—nor by doctors. A prominent English surgeon of the Middle Ages, Sir Charles Bell, could not "think of an operation without heart sickness," according to a contemporary biography. John Hunter, another famous physician of the day, "turned pale as death" before every operation. Not surprisingly, this state of affairs encouraged surgeons to work swiftly; seventeenth-century physician William Cheselden could remove a kidney stone in less than a minute, and Napoleon's surgeon once performed 200 amputations during a single battle.

But if surgery was traumatic for surgeons, the view from the other side of the scalpel was even worse. Here's how a nineteenth-century physician, who had undergone an operation himself, described the surgery patient's frame of mind before the discovery of anesthetics:

> Before the days of anaesthetics a patient preparing for
> an operation was like a condemned criminal preparing for

an execution. He counted the days till the appointed hour came. He listened for the echo in the street of the surgeon's carriage. He watched for his pull at the door bell, for his foot on the stair, for his step in the room, for the production of his dreaded instruments, for his few grave words and his last preparations before beginning; and then he surrendered his liberty and, revolting at the necessity, submitted to be held or bound, and helplessly gave up to the cruel knife.

Contrast this scenario with the typical surgical patient's experience today, and it becomes obvious just how amazing has been the progress of the last century and a half. Even for emergency surgery, where the patient can be rendered unconscious in a matter of minutes, the operation itself is utterly painless. This is a fact of modern medicine that's often taken for granted, but without anesthesia there could be no heart transplants, no coronary-artery bypass surgery, no cataract removal, no nose jobs or gallbladder removals. It's not just that these operations would be almost unbearably painful; they would be too lengthy and delicate for even the most skillful surgeon to perform on a screaming and writhing patient. Thus, the most wondrous thing about anesthesia is not the pain it spares us (though that would be wonder enough), but the countless lives it saves by making possible modern surgical techniques.

Anesthesia Rediscovered

Surgery did not emerge from the Dark Ages until the late date of 1842, when nitrous oxide was first used as an anesthetic in its now-familiar setting, the dentist's office.

Nitrous oxide is a simple chemical; each molecule is made up of one atom of oxygen and two of nitrogen. British chemist Joseph Priestly had discovered this gas in 1776, and soon its strange effects on the mind had earned it the nickname "laughing gas." In 1799 Humphry Davy announced that nitrous oxide could eliminate pain, and he suggested that it be used for this purpose in surgery. But in an oversight that would for nearly half a century condemn patients to indescribable suffering, doctors of the day dismissed the drug as an impractical means of anesthetizing patients.

Thus denied its rightful place in medicine, laughing gas became nothing more than a parlor amusement and road-show curiosity. It was at just such a traveling lecture, in Hartford, Connecticut, on December 10, 1844, that it came to the attention of an American dentist by the name of Horace Wells.

The promoter of the lecture, a chemist by the name of Colton, had a keen sense of drama and salesmanship, and in the days before the lecture he circulated flyers throughout the city promising a "Grand Exhibition of the effects of Nitrous Oxid [sic], Exhilarating or Laughing Gas!" In an advertising ploy that would have done P. T. Barnum proud, he announced that "Eight Strong Men are engaged to occupy the front seats to protect those under the influence of the Gas from injuring themselves or others." But, the flyer suggested, "probably no one will attempt to fight."

Of course, a fight very nearly *did* break out. A volunteer named Cooley inhaled the gas and promptly jumped off the stage to attack one of the strong men, who just as promptly fled. Cooley followed at full tilt, jumped over a chair, tripped, and fell to the ground with a nasty gash on his leg.

Sitting in the audience was Hartford dentist Horace Wells. He questioned Cooley after the lecture and learned that the young clerk had felt no pain at the time of the injury.

Intrigued, Wells guessed that nitrous oxide might be useful to relieve the pain of tooth extractions (fortunately he wasn't aware of the fact that the doctors had dismissed such a possibility decades before), obtained a quantity of gas from the lecturer, and set out to test its effectiveness in dentistry.

Wells set up a freewheeling experiment with himself as the subject. He inhaled the gas until he felt its effects coming on, at which time a colleague, Dr. Riggs, pulled out one of his teeth. According to Riggs's account of the operation, the tooth was a stubborn one and did not come out easily, but Wells never complained. When the effects of the gas wore off, Wells swung his hands in the air and proclaimed, in what may have been the understatement of the century, "a new era in tooth-pulling."

Soon Wells began using this wondrous gas in his dental practice, publicizing it at every opportunity. It wasn't long before he recognized the broader implications of his discovery, and he was soon busy demonstrating the effects of nitrous oxide to other doctors. In January 1845 he arranged a demonstration at Massachusetts General Hospital, but it did not go well; the patient awoke too soon and began screaming in pain.

This setback nearly sent nitrous oxide back to the carnival tents, and it subjected Wells to ridicule. It was not until twenty years later that nitrous oxide was again popularized by the same lecturer who'd given Wells his original sample. By the late 1860s, it was a mainstay of dentistry, and it has been ever since.

Ether and the "Death of Pain"

Just as with nitrous oxide, the introduction of ether into the medical world was not a true discovery but a rediscovery. The gas was discovered in 1540; it was named "aether" in 1730, and its properties were described in 1818 by Michael Faraday, the famous British chemist and student of Davy, who noted that its effects were "similar to those occasioned by nitrous oxide." Just as with nitrous oxide, however, the possibility of using ether for surgery was dismissed because of the mistaken belief that it was too dangerous.

The honor for the first use of ether in medicine goes to Georgia physician Crawford W. Long, who in March 1842 had a friend inhale the gas while Long removed a tumor from his neck. But Long never published his findings, and it remained for one of Wells's former dental assistants to bring ether to the attention of the medical world.

His name was William T. G. Morton, the place was, once again, Massachusetts General Hospital, and the date was October 16, 1846. The event is one of the watersheds of modern medicine, ranking alongside such events as Fleming's discovery of penicillin and Christiaan Barnard's first heart transplant.

Remarkably, Morton was not a physician at the time, but a medical student. He was also, however, a practicing dentist, and had learned a great deal about nitrous oxide from his former associate, Wells. His interest in nitrous oxide eventually led him to experiment with ether. He practiced on his pet spaniel and on cats, hens, rats, friends, and finally himself. He successfully—but without great fanfare—used it for a tooth extraction.

Finally, when all was ready, he prepared to announce his discovery to the medical community of Boston. His approach was very different than that of Wells. Aware of the great significance of the event, he took pains to ensure that it—and he—would receive the proper attention. He asked Harvard professor J. C. Warren for permission to try ether in a well-publicized operation; Warren agreed and scheduled the experiment for October 16.

Of course, the story that a second-year medical student had solved one of the greatest problems in medicine attracted a lot of attention, and on the morning of the 16th, the gallery was packed with the greatest medical minds of Boston—most of them full of skepticism. Edward Gilbert Abbott, a young man with a tumor on his neck, was the patient; Dr. Warren was the surgeon.

Initial preparations did not take long, for this was 1846 and the advent of sterile operating rooms, hand-scrubbing, and surgical gowns and masks were still in the future. At 9 A.M., Dr. Warren was ready, dressed in formal morning clothes; the patient lay ready, though perhaps not entirely willing, in an open shirt and plain black trousers. A team of strong men to hold down the patient—a standard part of a surgical team of the day—stood by.

But where was Morton? Minutes passed; then more. The buzzing of the skeptics in the gallery grew louder; the surgeon grew impatient. Finally he took his scalpel in hand and announced that he would wait no longer. Turning to the patient, he prepared to cut.

Just then Morton rushed in, explaining that he'd been delayed by the need to put some finishing touches on the apparatus he'd devised to administer the ether. The surgeon stepped aside, and Morton set to work beneath the cold smiles of the skeptical audience.

Within five minutes his patient was unconscious. The patient lay quietly as Dr. Warren worked. The strong men stood idle; the skeptics grew quiet. When he was done, the surgeon turned to his astonished colleagues in the gallery and announced, "Gentlemen, this is no humbug."

This pronouncement spread like wildfire. Doctors who hadn't witnessed this historic event were at first inclined to doubt it, but other demonstrations soon followed. Within a year, the esteemed medical professor Oliver Wendell Holmes, Sr., was telling his Harvard students that "the fierce extremity of suffering has been steeped in the waters of forgetfulness, and the deepest furrow in the knotted brow of agony has been smoothed forever."

Thus did a single operation on an autumn day in Boston transform the entire discipline of surgery. What had been a collection of limited, often last-ditch efforts dreaded by patients and doctors alike was suddenly transformed into a medical specialty that could work wonders. Soon surgeons were performing operations that would have been impossible just a few years earlier and were learning far more about the workings of the human body than had centuries of predecessors. And it was ether, the sweet-smelling, colorless gas once dismissed so casually as a mere curiosity, that first opened the door to new techniques which eventually led to today's mind-boggling advances in surgery and high-technology medicine.

In 1896, poet-physician Weir Mitchell anticipated the debt that the future physicians would owe Morton and his wondrous gas; in a poem celebrating the 50th anniversary of the discovery of ether anesthesia, he wrote:

> Whatever triumphs still shall hold the mind,
> Whatever gift shall yet enrich mankind,
> Ah! here no hour shall strike through all the years,
> No hour as sweet, as when hope, doubt, and fears,
> 'Mid deepening stillness, watched one eager brain,
> With Godlike will, decree the Death of Pain.

The Pioneers of Anesthesia: A Tragic Postscript

Fame is not always kind. For many of the players involved, the events surrounding the discovery of anesthetics were the beginning not of happiness and prosperity, but of lifelong misery and despair.

Take William Morton, for instance. Acting on others' advice, he applied for a patent for ether in 1846. Allegations of improprieties surrounding his patent application soon followed, as did legal challenges by his old dental associate Horace Wells, his former chemistry professor Charles T. Jackson, and the Georgian physician Crawford Long. Wells, feeling that the introduction of ether unfairly stole the spotlight from his own discovery of nitrous oxide and its anesthetic properties, eventually lost his sanity and committed suicide; Jackson also fell victim to insanity, while Morton himself eventually died in poverty and misery, the victim of apoplexy.

And what of Edward Gilbert Abbott, the patient at Morton's famous demonstration of ether? Orphaned at the age of eleven, he had grown up in poverty and suffered from mysterious and recurrent illnesses throughout his life. Perhaps it was in search of their cause that he came to Massachusetts General Hospital in late September 1846, seeking treatment at the age of 21 for a tumor on the left side of his neck.

In an article in the *New England Journal of Medicine,* physicians Leroy D. Vandam and John Adams Abbott (the latter a distant relative of Edward Gilbert Abbott and, until he retired, a physician at Mass. General) question whether the operation was necessary at all; they note that the tumor did not seem to be cancerous, was not enlarged, did not seem to create discomfort, did not affect Abbott's speech, and was not unduly offensive in appearance—in fact, it was not the sort of growth that would normally be removed in those days.

Was Abbott kept at the hospital for three weeks and counseled to undergo an operation simply so that he could serve as a subject for Morton's demonstration? Perhaps we shall never know, but Vandam and Abbott believe it was possible.

After the operation, Edward Abbott spent nearly another two months in the hospital. According to the hospital record, he was discharged on December 7 with "genl health m. improved," but with his tumor the same size as it had been before the operation!

For a while, his fortune improved; he advanced in the printing trade and eventually became an assistant editor of the *Boston Herald,* and, after that, the editor and owner of the *Cambridge Mercury,* a short-lived paper whose main purpose was to oppose newly enacted temperance laws.

On November 27, 1855, less than ten years after his celebrated operation, Edward Gilbert Abbott died of tuberculosis. Although anesthesia was already transforming the practice of medicine, Abbott's death attracted little public notice. Even the *Boston Herald,* for which he had once worked, did not record his death until four days later. Here's how this pioneer patient from the dawn of anesthesia was remembered that day, in the words of the obituary itself:

DEATH OF A PRINTER

Edward G. Abbott well-known printer and editor died at Maplewood, Malden on Tuesday of consumption. He was thirty years of age and leaves a widow and two children.

Chloroform: Royal Anesthetic or "Decoy of Satan"?

The next advance in anesthesia was the discovery of chloroform. A Scottish gynecologist, Dr. James Young Simpson, had been impressed with ether's effects, but found it unsuitable for much of his gynecological work. He set out to investigate other gases, and a contemporary account of how he and his team of "investigators" discovered chloroform stands in contrast to the sophisticated and multimillion-dollar research programs of modern pharmaceutical companies. A colleague of Simpson's described the historic events thusly:

> Late one evening—it was the 4th of November 1847—on returning home after a weary day's work, Dr. Simpson, with his two friends and assistants Drs. Keith and Duncan, sat down to their somewhat hazardous work in Dr. Simpson's dining room. Having inhaled several substances, but without much effect, it occurred to Dr. Simpson to try a ponderous material which he had formerly set aside on a lumber table, and which on account of its great weight, he had hitherto regarded as of no likelihood whatever. *That* happened to be a small bottle of chloroform. It was searched for and recovered from beneath a heap of waste paper. And with each tumbler newly charged the inhalers resumed their vocation. Immediately an unwonted hilarity seized the party; they became bright-eyed, very happy and very loquacious—expatiating on the delicious aroma of the new fluid. The conversation was of unusual intelligence and quite charmed the listeners. . . .
>
> But suddenly there was talk of sounds being heard like those of a cotton mill, louder and louder; a moment more and then all was quiet—and then *crash*. The inhaling party slipped off their chairs and flopped on to the floor unconscious.

Within two weeks, Simpson had begun to use his new discovery in his obstetrical practice, and obtained excellent results. In chloroform he believed that he had found at last a solution to the age-old problem of painful childbirth, and he enthusiastically began promoting its use.

But Simpson was a better judge of chemistry than he was of human nature. Suddenly, he found his wonder drug attacked from an unlikely source: the pulpit. Ministers denounced chloroform as a "decoy of Satan"; it violated, they claimed, God's ancient edict to Eve: "In sorrow thou shalt bring forth children." Simpson countered Scripture with Scripture: "And the Lord God caused a deep sleep to fall upon Adam, and he slept; and he took one of his ribs and closed up the flesh instead thereof."

In the end, the matter was resolved not by divine intervention but by royal action, when Queen Victoria used chloroform for the birth of her seventh child. Even so, critics were not immediately swayed; even the prestigious medical journal *Lancet* warned that "in no case could it be justifiable to administer chloroform in a perfectly ordinary labour."

Evidently the Queen's physician did not agree; four years later Victoria received chloroform for the birth of her next child. Finally, with this two-time vote of approval, the "decoy of Satan" began to flourish, and soon became popularized as "anesthesia à la Reine"—the Queen's anesthesia.

Anesthesia Today: Spectacular Benefits— and Profound Dangers

Today, of course, anesthesia is a cornerstone of medicine. Ether and chloroform are obsolete, supplanted by safer drugs. Nitrous oxide remains one of the most widely used anesthetics for dentistry and minor operations; combined with other anesthetics, it's used in major surgery as well. The branch of medicine known as anesthesiology involves sophisticated and expensive equipment and years of training, and is served by dozens of scientific journals and publications.

The reason for all the attention lavished on anesthetics is simple: they are potentially the most dangerous drugs of all. General anesthetics do more than block pain; they drive a chemical wedge between the body and the parts of the brain that normally serve to protect it. An anesthetized patient can literally suffocate under the anesthesiologist's nose and never stir or struggle—indeed, never give an outward sign at all until it's too late. His gag reflex—which is nature's way of keeping harmful foreign material out of the lungs and breathing passages—disappears, and if he should vomit, corrosive digestive juices can quickly sear his lungs and kill him. A patient under general anesthesia can lapse into a coma with no outward sign other than a change in the size of his pupils. Under these circumstances, the only thing standing between the patient and tragedy is the vigilance of the anesthesiologist. More than any other kind of doctor, he holds his patients' lives in his hands. It is an awesome responsibility.

And yet the most surprising thing about these potent drugs is their track record for safety. Despite their inherent dangers, only rarely do any problems arise. Every day, surgeons perform thousands and thousands of operations under general anesthesia. They remove diseased gallbladders, stitch up injured organs, bypass clogged arteries, and cut away infections and tumors. They insert stainless steel hips, Teflon-coated heart valves, artificial blood vessels made of woven Dacron, kidneys, livers, hearts, and corneas—all routinely. The occasional incidents where something goes wrong are tragic, and likely to end up on the front page of a local paper or in court. But the publicity surrounding these events tends to obscure how rare they really are. And while it's true that general anesthesia should be avoided when it's unnecessary (as is true of any medical treatment), for patients needing surgery the benefits far outweigh the risks.

Today, anesthesiologists have a whole range of anesthetics at their disposal (see the Quick Reference for an overview of modern anesthetics), and they spend years learning how to use these drugs safely and effectively. And yet, paradoxically, doctors' understanding of how these drugs work is little better today than it was in the time of Wells, Morton, and Simpson. Various theories focus on lipids, biochemistry, the surface tension of cells, and other possible mechanisms of action, but no theory offers an entirely satisfactory explanation. Despite the central role that they play in modern medicine, these drugs remain, in their essence, as mysterious and wondrous as they did to the incredulous audiences attending Colton's "Grand Exhibition" nearly a century and a half ago.

Analgesics

Analgesics, like anesthetics, are used to reduce or block pain. But they're more focused than both general anesthetics, which block consciousness altogether, and local anesthetics, which block *all* sensation in the affected part of the body. The boundaries between these categories are a little fuzzy; nitrous oxide, for example, is technically an analgesic, but it's usually grouped with the anesthetics because it's often used in combination with them during general anesthesia. Steroids, too, are painkillers of sorts—they're especially useful for itching rashes and pain caused by inflammation—but their pain-relief qualities are secondary, a result of their ability to clear up the rash or inflammation itself.

Nonetheless, the term "analgesics" usually refers to the drugs we often think of as painkillers: narcotics, aspirin and related compounds, acetaminophen (Tylenol®, for example), and nonsteroidal antiinflammatory drugs (Motrin®, Nuprin™, Advil™, and several other brands of ibuprofen, for example).

Narcotics

We took an in-depth look at narcotics and how they work in the last chapter. There's only one additional point we should make about them here: they are not entirely deserving of their bad reputation. It is true that they have a great potential for abuse, but often overlooked is the fact that after thousands of years they remain the most effective painkillers ever discovered. And the stories of patients who entered a hospital for an operation and came out an addict are, for the most part, just that: stories. In fact, for patients in hospitals the problem is likely to be the *underuse,* rather than overuse, of narcotics.

Addiction of hospital patients almost never occurs; one estimate is that it occurs among burn patients (who routinely receive large doses of narcotics over extended periods of time) in only about one case in a thousand. And even when it does occur, this type of addiction is almost always easily cured, since the underlying social and psychological forces that lead to addiction on the street are absent.

Panic and Pain

Why do people turn their heads away before they get a shot? Why does an unexpected injury seem less painful than if we'd known it was coming? Why do postsurgical patients on a fixed schedule of narcotics require more pain relief than patients who know they can have painkillers on demand? Why does pain make it so difficult to think clearly and rationally? Why do women in childbirth report feeling "schizy" as they approach transition, the most painful part of labor? Recent research has revealed that there may be a biochemical answer to all of these questions and more.

The underlying reason for all of these phenomena lies with the brain's neurotransmitter system, which we looked at in detail in Chapter 6. The evidence suggests that pain, panic, and psychosis all share the same neurological pathway within the brain. When pain signals travel along this path, our brains correctly interpret

---

them and register both pain and the emotions that go along with it (such as rage and fear). In psychosis a false alarm seems to travel along the path; the victim feels no physical pain, but does feel many of the same emotions that would ordinarily accompany it. It's as if he or she experiences pain without actually feeling it. Similarly, the often-observed fact that schizophrenics don't feel pain may be caused by these same pathways being crowded with false signals, in effect jamming the pain signals.

There's some easily seen circumstantial evidence that also supports this view. For instance, patients suffering from severe, unrelenting pain exhibit many of the symptoms usually associated with psychosis and panic—fear, anxiety, rage, and confusion. Further evidence of the link between panic and pain comes from reports of patients receiving narcotics for pain: They report that they still feel the pain, but it does not "bother" them. Also, researchers have found that methadone—a narcotic related to morphine and heroin—can sometimes reduce the symptoms of mania, depressive psychosis, depression, and paranoid schizophrenia.

The implications of all this are only just beginning to be explored, and eventually they may lead to a new understanding of both pain and psychosis—and new treatments for each of them. Already, for example, it's been suggested that narcotics may be useful for treating some forms of psychosis (in years past they were put to just such a use, but with the advent of chlorpromazine and other antipsychotics doctors abandoned them for treatment of psychosis and depression). In fact, there is support for the thesis that narcotics actually *help* some "addicts" by helping to control psychotic symptoms—in other words, that some people abuse narcotics not to get high but simply to keep from feeling bad.

These discoveries also suggest that effective analgesia may depend on controlling pain's *emotional* aspects as much as or more than its *physical* aspects. Assuming this to be so, we may see greater use of, say, antianxiety drugs to augment the effectiveness of painkillers. Also, the implications go beyond pharmacology; this evidence helps us understand why certain nonchemical means of reducing pain can be so effective. Giving patients control over their narcotics, for example, can help reduce their anxiety and fear of pain and thus function as a sort of nonchemical narcotic; similarly, relaxation exercises for childbirth give women in labor a powerful tool for reducing the emotional aspects of the pain they experience.

In contrast to the largely theoretical risk of hospital addiction are studies showing that many doctors and nurses tend to undermedicate their patients who are in pain. Doctors write medication orders with dosages too low to be effective, or write orders for nurses to dispense narcotics "as needed." Nurses, in turn, tend to interpret these orders with caution, with needless suffering often the result. For nurses and physicians alike, the reasons for such undue caution are many—lack of a realistic understanding of the likelihood of addiction, an irrational dislike of narcotics, a misunderstanding of how they are best administered. Narcotics are most effective, for example, if they're given *before* the pain starts to get severe. A major factor seems to be the subjective nature of pain. There are no precise laboratory tests that can reliably determine the amount of pain a patient suffers from, and so the only guidelines are the patient's perceptions. These may vary considerably from one patient to another (there seems to be some physiological truth to the idea that different people have different "thresholds of pain"); also, persons from different ethnic backgrounds tend to react to pain in very different ways, making it hard for nurses to assess the amount of pain they actually feel (studies have revealed, for instance, that Italians and Jews are more vocal about their pain than, say, Irish or English patients).

The solution to this dilemma is surprisingly simple. *The proper level of narcotic painkillers is best determined by the patient's own perceptions.* There are some practical constraints, of course, such as those imposed by narcotics' side effects. But for most patients and in most circumstances, the patient is the best judge, and the idea that he or she won't be able to make responsible judgments regarding pain relief just doesn't hold water. In fact, knowing that one has control over one's painkillers seems, in and of itself, to help control pain; research has shown that patients permitted to receive narcotics on demand actually require less of them than patients tied to fixed doses and schedules.

Children and Narcotics

If the underuse of narcotics is a problem for adults, it is even more so for children. A study reported by A. K. Jacox in the book *Pain: A Source Book for Nurses and Other Health Professionals* (Little, Brown, 1977) looked at 25 children who underwent major surgery in a large teaching hospital. More than half received no painkillers at all at *any* time during their hospitalization—this

144

despite the fact that orders for analgesics had been written in 21 of the cases. One six-year-old boy had undergone 13 operations over a number of years, and had received painkillers only once in all that time.

Why is this needless suffering inflicted on children? The problem is largely one of myths and misperceptions among health care workers. Researchers Elan and Anderson, for example, identify seven "old nurses' tales" that often lead to inadequate pain relief in children:

1. *Children have immature nervous systems, and thus experience pain with less intensity than adults.* The neurologic theory underlying this view has been discredited both by new discoveries and by clinical experience. Elan and Anderson point out, for example, that a routine circumcision offers plenty of evidence that newborns perceive and respond to pain. (And yet pain medication is rarely given for circumcisions!)

2. *Children recover more quickly than adults.* Even if this statement is true—and that in itself is arguable—so what? Pain is pain, whether it lasts for a day or a week.

3. *Children who receive narcotics will become addicted.* The truth is that children recovering from operations will likely receive narcotics for only a few days at most—far too short a time for addiction to develop. In addition, there are other instances in which the fear of addiction makes no sense whatsoever. For example, the researchers spoke with a group of nurses who felt guilty because a terminally ill eight-year-old was addicted to narcotics, even though they acknowledged that the alternative was severe pain. And even in nonterminal cases where addiction might occur—in burn units, for instance—it can be overcome later by gradually reducing the doses of narcotics.

4. *Narcotics are dangerous because they lower the rate of breathing in children.* True, but no more so than among adults when dosages are calculated according to body weight.

5. *Children can't tell you where they hurt.* In fact, children *can* tell you where they hurt, and with great accuracy. Even children as young as four years old are almost always able to correctly place an "X" on a body chart indicating where they feel pain.

6. *Children hate nurses who give them injections.* This may be so, but it's no excuse to withhold pain medication. A great deal depends on the nurse's attitude; the child's terror can be soothed to some extent by answering his or her questions, explaining the need for and purpose of the injection, and, above all, remaining calm and supportive. And while nobody enjoys playing the heavy, the nurse's primary obligation is to provide care for the patient—not to be liked. Certainly nobody would use this rationale to deny, say, a shot

of penicillin to a child who needed it. This "nurses' tale" is reinforced by another, related one:

7. *Narcotics, to be effective, must be given by a painful injection.* Not always; if a child already has an intravenous line for other medications, painkillers can sometimes be given through this line, avoiding the need for an injection. Once the child can tolerate solid food, he or she may be able to take oral painkillers.

Aspirin: The Willow Bark Wonder

What would a medicine chest be without aspirin? These unassuming white tablets are as much a part of modern life as telephones, automobiles, and the light bulb. And yet like them, aspirin has been around only since the last half of the last century. For the thousands of years before, mankind had at its disposal only those painkillers known since prehistoric times.

The story of aspirin and its descendants is still in the making, for as we've studied more and more about this remarkable drug, we've gained deeper insights into not only pain but a vast array of processes occurring in the human body. The payoff has already begun, with a flurry of new drugs introduced in recent years that for many patients offer either better pain relief or fewer side effects than aspirin itself. Future research promises even bigger breakthroughs, for we are finding that aspirin and related drugs affect substances within the body that help regulate not only pain and fever, but also such diverse activities as kidney function, digestion, pregnancy, and childbirth. Thus, it's anyone's guess as to where current investigations will lead, and what new uses will be found for aspirin and related drugs along the way (see box).

Aspirin, Strokes, and Heart Attacks

It's said that you can't teach an old dog new tricks, but that truism doesn't always hold true in the pharmaceutical world. In recent years scientists have found that their old friend aspirin has a few tricks up its sleeve when it comes to heart disease and strokes.

First came the discovery, in the early 1970s, that aspirin helps prevent strokes. Strokes occur when the blood flow to the brain is interrupted, usually because of clogged arteries. Often there occurs before a stroke one or more *transient ischemic attacks* (TIAs), which may appear minutes, hours, days, weeks, or months before a stroke, and which consist of strokelike symptoms—dizziness, loss of consciousness, tingling or even paralysis—that appear and then go away. After the TIA is over, the person usually is fine, with no symptoms remaining from the attack.

Doctors have long understood the physiological reason for these seemingly mysterious attacks. They are to the brain what angina is to the heart: evidence that something is interfering with the supply of blood—usually because the artery is partially clogged or constricted (see Chapter 5). Blood may be able to get through an artery that's only partially clogged, but if, say, blood pressure drops, the blood supply may be temporarily reduced or cut off. The part of the brain served by this blood supply then becomes starved for oxygen and begins to malfunction, leading to the symptoms of TIA.

Even though TIAs are ominous, there's a positive side to them. *If* a person recognizes a TIA for what it is (unfortunately, TIAs are often dismissed as nothing more than symptoms of old age by those who experience them), and *if* there's time to seek medical attention, it may be possible to avoid a stroke.

One means of doing just that became apparent in 1978, when the results of a Canadian study were published in the *New England Journal of Medicine*. The authors of the article had discovered that for patients who'd suffered TIAs, aspirin helped prevent subsequent strokes. The results were more than just good; they were amazing: the mortality rate in the group receiving aspirin was cut by approximately 50 percent. (Curiously, this effect is only apparent in men; aspirin seems to have no effect on strokes in women.)

Equally impressive results have since been obtained for heart patients. A recent study conducted in Veterans Administration hospitals showed that for patients with unstable angina—the kind of angina most likely to lead to a heart attack—low daily doses of aspirin again reduced the death rate by half. Surprisingly, the beneficial effects continued even after discontinuation of the aspirin regimen; a year later the death rate was 43 percent lower for patients who'd taken the aspirin.

The VA study and others suggest that *low* doses of aspirin are best for preventing heart attacks and strokes. Researchers think they know why. It seems that aspirin interferes with the manufacture of certain substances in the body that regulate clotting. These two substances, *thromboxane* and *prostacyclin*, are chemically related to the prostaglandins that cause pain, fever, and inflammation. Each has opposing effects on the blood, and proper clotting depends on keeping them in balance. Thromboxane promotes clotting and causes arteries to constrict (become tighter), while prostacyclin prevents clot formation and relaxes arteries. Ordinary doses of aspirin prevent the formation of both thromboxane and prostacyclin, but low doses—a fourth of a tablet a day or less—seem to affect thromboxane while leaving prostacyclin relatively unaffected. Thus they help prevent the clotting that can lead to both angina and strokes.

Researchers have only begun to study the potential role of aspirin in the treatment and prevention of these and other cardiovascular disorders. But if subsequent studies support the results of the VA study, ordinary aspirin may well turn out to be one of our most important and versatile wonder drugs in years to come.

This remarkable story began in the last half of the nineteenth century. Scientists were looking for a fever-reducing drug to replace quinine, which was both scarce and expensive. The search led to the *salicylates,* a group of chemicals derived from the bark of the willow tree.

The *antipyretic*—that is, fever-reducing—properties of willow bark have been known since ancient times, but the active ingredient *salicin* was not discovered until 1827. In 1838 *salicylic acid,* the first salicylate to be used for medicinal purposes, was made from salicyn, but it proved suitable for external use only. *Sodium salicylate* was the first of the group to be used internally; the year was 1875 and the disease was rheumatic fever. *Phenyl salicylate* followed in 1886 and *acetylsalicylic acid*—aspirin—in 1899.

Aspirin is not the only salicylate in use today, but it remains the most popular and is usually the most effective. It has three basic actions—antipyretic, analgesic, and antiinflammatory—which together make it one of the most versatile and useful drugs available. On top of its effectiveness, aspirin has several other features that make it a doctor's dream come true. It doesn't cause drowsiness, depression, euphoria, or other changes in consciousness and shows no tendency to create addiction or tolerance to its effects.

There are some limiting factors, of course. A small percentage of people are allergic to aspirin and break out in a rash or hives when they take it. Aspirin can be hard on the stomach and shouldn't be taken by people with ulcers or other stomach problems. In high doses it interferes with the blood's ability to clot and can aggravate kidney disease. Overdoses damage the liver and can be fatal.

For children, overdose is a particular problem. Aspirin is the most common cause of poisoning in children. The problem is not so much the drug's toxicity as the fact that children's aspirin is likely to be around and often looks and tastes like candy. Another problem with children and aspirin is an apparent link between the drug and Reye's syndrome, a frightening and often fatal children's disorder characterized by seizures and other symptoms. Studies suggest that Reye's syndrome is more frequent in children who have taken aspirin while suffering from chickenpox or flu, and although the studies aren't conclusive, they've led doctors to suggest acetaminophen (see below) for the treatment of fever in young children.

However, with the exception of children's overdose, serious adverse reactions to aspirin occur only very rarely. And stomach problems can be minimized with *enteric-coated* aspirin, which have a special coating to contain the aspirin while it travels through the sensitive stomach. The enteric coating permits the aspirin to dissolve in the small intestine, where it's much less likely to cause nausea or other gastrointestinal disturbances. And for patients who, because of ulcers, poor kidney function, or allergies can't tolerate aspirin, there are two widely used alternatives: acetaminophen and nonsteroidal antiinflammatory drugs (NSAIDs).

Acetaminophen

Acetaminophen (Tylenol®, Datril®, Panadol®, Anacin-3®) is the most widely used alternative to aspirin. Its properties are identical to aspirin's in most respects, but it's easier on the stomach and less likely to cause an allergic reaction.

On the downside, it lacks aspirin's antiinflammatory properties, which makes it unsuitable for treatment of arthritis. Also, overdoses (for example, 50 extra-strength tablets) can cause death from liver failure. There is also some evidence—though it is disputed by acetaminophen manufacturers—that therapeutic doses of acetaminophen may cause less extensive liver damage. According to an editorial in the *Journal of the American Medical Association,* serious liver damage has resulted from long-term use of as few as six extra-strength tablets a day. Of course, such occurrences are very rare, and since acetaminophen doesn't help arthritis (the primary indication for long-term use of aspirin), the drug is less likely to be used in high doses or for lengthy periods of time. Nonetheless, these findings do suggest that where relief is needed for chronic pain, aspirin may be a better choice.

In one of those coincidences that seem to occur so frequently in the history of pharmacy, acetaminophen was discovered by the same Alsatian chemist, Charles-Frederick Gerhardt, who would discover aspirin a year later. It is a derivative of a chemical known as *para-aminophenol*. Other derivatives of this chemical, such as phenacetin and acetanilide, share acetaminophen's analgesic and antipyretic properties, but acetaminophen is the least toxic member of the family. (Acetanilide's toxicity led to its abandonment in favor of phenacetin in the late 1800s; today, phenacetin is all but abandoned as well.)

NSAIDS

The nonsteroidal antiinflammatory drugs—known as NSAIDs—are the newest members of the analgesic community, and they've received a great deal of attention lately, both from the public and from pharmaceutical houses. *Ibuprofen* (Motrin®, Nuprin®, Advil®) is perhaps the best known, since it has recently become available in nonprescription form, but all of them have similar pharmacologic properties. Millions of arthritis patients have used ibuprofen (under the brand name Motrin®) for its ability to relieve pain and reduce inflammation of arthritic joints. But though its FDA approval originally applied only to arthritis, the drug gained popularity as a remedy for menstrual cramps. Now, in the form of such over-the-counter products as Nuprin® and Advil®, it's being promoted as a "new" alternative to other analgesics for aches and pains of all descriptions.

But does this widely touted wonder drug really work any better than aspirin? Not really. Like acetaminophen, it's easier on the stomach than aspirin, and so it may be an attractive alternative for arthritis patients who can't tolerate aspirin (remember that acetaminophen isn't effective against the inflammation of arthritis). However, people who are allergic to aspirin shouldn't take ibuprofen (or any other NSAID). As far as its effectiveness, a number of studies indicate that aspirin and ibuprofen work about equally well for relief of pain and inflammation.

Of course, that in itself is a pretty impressive performance, because *nothing* has been found to beat aspirin for the relief of mild to moderate pain. Even such narcotics as propoxyphene (Darvon®), oxycodone (Percodan®), and codeine can't beat it for ordinary garden-variety pain of, say, a headache or twisted ankle. (The advantage of these drugs comes into play when more severe pain is involved. Unlike aspirin, their pain-relieving properties increase as dosage increases, so doctors can prescribe larger doses when necessary. With aspirin, acetaminophen, and NSAIDs, by contrast, there's a "ceiling" beyond which higher doses don't provide more pain relief).

Wonder Drugs That Weren't: Oraflex

In April 1982, the pharmaceutical firm of Eli Lilly announced a revolution in medicine. After nearly a century, aspirin had finally been toppled as the most effective antiarthritis medication by a newcomer: benoxaprofen (Oraflex®). According to Eli Lilly Co., which manufactured the drug, Oraflex was a "new direction in antiarthritic therapy" that had been "well accepted" in a number of European countries. According to one expert, it was "much more potent a painkiller than aspirin . . . you can take it in large quantities and there's no gastrointestinal bleeding . . . and most miraculous of all, benoxaprofen seems to actually reverse the joint damage caused by arthritis inflammation." Within three weeks of its introduction, sales of Oraflex had reached $1.3 million and were still climbing.

Then, in May 1982—just weeks after this successful launch—reports from Britain began documenting side effects and even deaths related to this "miracle" drug. By August the drug had been outlawed in Britain and withdrawn from the American market. In two years of use in the United Kingdom, the drug had caused at least 4,000 adverse reactions and 96 deaths. In many cases the cause of death was, ironically, gastrointestinal bleeding and perforated ulcers. In others, liver and kidney damage were responsible.

Later, evidence came to light showing that Lilly was aware of these problems even before the drug was introduced in the United States, but had failed to report them to the FDA. Lilly officials insist that they did nothing wrong; the European deaths were to be "expected" from a drug such as Oraflex, they said.

Late in 1983, Lilly notified the few physicians still authorized to prescribe Oraflex that it had been associated with an increased incidence of cancer in experiments with mice and instructed the doctors to stop prescribing the drug immediately. In a little more than a year and a half, the "miracle" of Oraflex had proved to be a bust. In fact, the miracle was almost entirely in the marketing, for there was no convincing evidence that Oraflex was more effective than aspirin or that it reversed joint damage caused by arthritis.

Together, the drugs discussed in this section give you a useful range of alternatives for relief of pain, fever, and inflammation. Most doctors still consider aspirin the drug of choice—*if* the patient can tolerate it—with acetaminophen and ibuprofen as good alternatives.

Prostaglandins and Pain: How Nonnarcotic Analgesics Work

As we saw in the last chapter, pain is ultimately controlled by the brain's neurotransmitter system, with endorphins (a type of narcotic manufactured by the brain) playing a central role. However, the signals that are translated into a sensation of pain usually originate elsewhere. Pain is nature's newspaper (or scandal sheet, if you prefer). It carries reports from the far reaches of the body into the brain, calling attention to the fact that things are amiss and that something needs to be done. Like any seasoned journalist, though, it knows how fickle and easily distracted the human mind is, and it isn't content merely to drop off the bad news and leave. It hangs around, spreading doom and gloom, until some sort of action is taken to resolve the problem.

Now, under ordinary circumstances, that's a pretty good system for keeping the body in top working order. But when we *can't* do anything about the reason for the pain—either because we don't understand or can't treat the cause—it becomes decidedly *un*useful. That's when we begin to rummage through the medicine cabinet for a painkiller.

Both aspirin and NSAIDs block unnecessary pain signals right at their source, by preventing the formation of substances known as *prostaglandins.* When we stub a toe or bite our tongue, two events occur that will influence our perception of pain. Almost immediately, a nerve impulse is sent to the brain informing us of our misfortune. At the same time, the cells near the injury begin to manufacture prostaglandins, which in turn activate pain receptors on nearby nerve cells. The prostaglandins don't actually *transmit* the pain signals; they simply turn the pain network on. Once this network is activated, it translates formerly nonpainful sensations into pain. (Think of a swollen toe, and how the slightest touch can cause daggerlike pain.)

By preventing the formation of prostaglandins, aspirin and NSAIDs help muffle this alarm system. They don't shut down prostaglandin production entirely, but they do reduce the amount that the body produces. However, these drugs have little effect on sudden, sharp pain sensations, which are sent directly to the brain and have little to do with prostaglandins; thus, if you were to take two aspirin and then fall down and bump your head, you'd most certainly feel pain. (Not so if you were anesthetized with, say, nitrous oxide; you'd be unaware of any pain until the effects wore off.)

Prostaglandins also get involved in inflammation; that's why pain and swelling so often go hand in hand. Animal experiments have shown that it's possible to simulate the inflammation of arthritis by injecting prostaglandins into a joint (any volunteers?), thus confirming the means by which aspirin helps relieve some of the symptoms of arthritis.

The action of acetaminophen is less well understood than aspirin and NSAIDs. It seems pretty clear that it also reduces the production of prostaglandins, but the fact that acetaminophen doesn't affect inflammation suggests that different prostaglandins are involved in pain and inflammation. Studies have also shown that acetaminophen is better than aspirin at inhibiting prostaglandin release in the brain itself, but less so for prostaglandins produced in the spleen. Exactly what all this means must await a fuller understanding of the complex role that prostaglandins play in the body, but these findings suggest that they interact in several different ways to regulate pain sensations.

Researchers are intensely interested in prostaglandins for more reasons than pain, though. As we suggested, the prostaglandins are a kind of chemical jack-of-all-trades within the body, with their role as gatekeepers of pain only one of an almost incredible variety of functions that they provide. They are present in almost every type of tissue and body fluid, and seem to have a regulatory role in virtually every function of the body.

That helps explain, for instance, why aspirin and related compounds reduce fever in addition to relieving pain. It seems that invading viruses and bacteria stimulate the release of prostaglandins in, among other places, the hypothalamus—a part of the brain that plays a key role in regulating various bodily processes. In the hypothalamus, prostaglandins help control the body's natural thermostat—known as the "set point" to doctors and biologists—which ordinarily keeps body temperature at or near 98.6 degrees Fahrenheit. These excess prostaglandins overstimulate the set point and thus cause fever. Once again, aspirin or one of its relatives comes to the rescue, blocking prostaglandin release and thereby lowering body temperature back toward normal. (Interestingly, these drugs won't lower the thermostat *below* 98.6 degrees, no matter how much of them you take.)

But don't get the impression that prostaglandins are all bad. In pregnant women, for instance, they trigger labor. The role of prostaglandins in labor, by the way, offers a hint as to why aspirin and NSAIDs are particularly effective for menstrual cramps. Prostaglandins help bring on labor by causing the smooth muscles of the uterus to contract. In nonpregnant women, the hormonal changes that occur during menstruation stimulate the release of prostaglandins, which in turn cause muscle spasms—that is, cramps—in the uterus. Thus, aspirin and NSAIDs do more than simply relieve the pain of these uterine cramps; they actually reduce or eliminate the cramps themselves.

Prostaglandins are even used as drugs in cases of congenital heart defects in newborn infants, where doctors use them to keep open the ductus arteriosus and thus buy time for lifesaving surgery. And this is only the beginning, for the incredible diversity of bodily functions in which prostaglandins figure suggest that synthetic prostaglandins may someday be among the most versatile and useful drugs ever developed. If those predictions come to pass, mankind will have traveled very far indeed along the journey that began with the bark of the willow tree.

8

To Be or Not to Be: Contraceptives and Fertility Drugs

Of all the wonders of the world, perhaps none is so mundane and yet miraculous as the birth of a child. Every day, infants are born by the millions—vast armies of innocents, crying for food and care in a world that has too little of both. The earth is inundated with children, far beyond the capacity of its people or governments to provide for them.

And yet the flood is not faceless. Each child is a brand-new attempt to perfect that most wondrous of creatures, man. Each shares the essential humanity of all who have gone before; each is kin to Abraham, Einstein, Caesar, and Buddha. To look upon the face of a sleeping child is to contemplate perfection, and to know that there is, after all, hope for our future.

All of this creates a profound paradox—a paradox that finds modern medicine at the center. There are, on the one hand, vast resources poured into the development of safe and effective contraceptives. There are physicians such as John Rock, who created the first contraceptive pill and believed until his dying day that it represented a way out of poverty and starvation for the Third World. At the same time, there are doctors whose life's work is devoted to doing everything they can to help bring more babies into the world—sometimes against the wishes of Mother Nature herself.

In this chapter, we'll be looking at the various drugs that can encourage or thwart reproduction. It's a topic that differs in many respects from others in this book, for it doesn't involve disease as such—at least not in the way that we usually think of disease. Pregnancy may entail pain, even risks, and most certainly requires medical attention, but it is after all a natural bodily process. Infertility is a malfunction of the reproductive system and can have devastating emotional effects, but it doesn't interfere with the body's ability to survive—and even thrive—in its environment.

Indeed, fertility and infertility are moral and social issues even more than they are medical ones, and these broader controversies have a greater impact on the use and acceptance of these drugs than do medical questions of safety and effectiveness.

The same is true in some other areas of medicine, of course; we have found time and again that as medicine moves beyond its traditional role of preventing and treating disease and takes on broader life-style problems, its mandate becomes less and less clear. Certainly there is no moral question over, say, a cure for cancer, but some might argue that, for instance, venereal diseases aren't all bad, since they might tend to discourage promiscuity—or, at least, that there are far worthier adversaries for medicine. And if these issues are controversial, what kind of furor could we expect to see over a "cure" for aggressiveness, or laziness? Or eccentricity, or political heresy? We have seen that road before, and as we look at some of the controversies surrounding contraception and fertility, we would do well to heed the lessons of the past.

The Pill

John Rock, a crusty New England obstetrician, was an unlikely candidate for the father of the sexual revolution. A world famous physician, and a devout Catholic and traditionalist, he once helped keep women out of Harvard Medical School because he believed that they weren't capable of being physicians. Better they should "stay at home and take care of their men and babies," he once said.

But in the mid-1950s, John Rock discovered a drug that would profoundly disrupt the traditional values he held so dear—a drug that came to be known simply as the Pill. Iron-ically, he had originally been looking for a way to *promote* fertility, not prevent it. But having discovered the Pill, he sensed that it might help slow a worldwide population explosion that threatened to devour the limited resources of the Third World. In developed nations, he thought that the Pill would be nothing more than a convenient way for married women to limit the size of their families, and he scoffed at the suggestion that it might find widespread use among the unmarried young women of America.

But even before the social upheaval of the 1960s, others were not so sure. When the FDA received a new drug applica-tion for the Pill in 1959, officials recognized the drug as a political hot potato and rejected the application. Searle, the pharmaceutical firm sponsoring Rock's research, appealed the denial, and Rock himself flew down to Washington to person-ally do battle with the bureaucrats of the FDA. He and the FDA did not quite come to blows over the appeal. When the young FDA doctor responsible for ruling on the appeal told him that he'd refer the issue to more experienced consultants, Rock grabbed him by the lapels and said, "You'll decide right now."

Caught between a Rock and a hard place, the FDA had no choice but to yield. Only months later, on May 11, 1960, the agency approved the Pill and—in the eyes of some, at least—launched the sexual revolution.

Rock believed that the Catholic Church could and would promote the use of the Pill in the Third World; the fact that it contained only natural hormones already present in women's bodies convinced him that it would win the Vatican's approval. What it did instead was to lead the Catholic Church to take a fresh look at its stand on contraception, with the result that it specifically banned Catholics from using any form of birth control other than abstinence. Since so much of the Third World is Catholic, this decree ruined Rock's hopes of stemming the worldwide population explosion in developing nations. But despite his differences with the Church, he remained a practic-ing Catholic until his death in 1984.

Meanwhile, in America things were not going according to Rock's vision, either. In 1962 Gloria Steinem declared the Pill "completely safe and effective" and proclaimed the emergence of the "autonomous girl"—a woman who "does not feel forced to choose between a career and marriage, and is therefore free to find fulfillment in a combination of the two." The world had changed, Steinem was saying; Hollywood screenwriters "should be warned that they can no longer build plots on loss of virginity or fainting pregnant heroines and expect to be believed." Even the world of etiquette was affected. One young woman wrote to Dear Abby asking whether a girl or her boyfriend should pay for the pills. (The girl, said Abby.)

Of course, the Pill was not solely responsible for the sexual revolution of the sixties. After all, other forms of contraception—diaphragms, condoms, foam, cream, and jelly—had been available for years, and even after the Pill there were still plenty of accidents. But as the symbol of an era, the Pill reigned supreme. Fundamentalists denounced it; feminists praised it. It was variously held responsible for everything from the corruption of youth to the emancipation of women.

As time went on, controversy over the Pill did not die down. In fact, as reports of problems with the Pill emerged—principally scientific studies showing an increased risk of disease among women who had taken it—new criticism came from many of its old champions. The Pill was not an emancipator of women, after all, they argued; it was actually a tool of oppression. Male researchers had created a drug that put women at risk while sparing their own gender and filling the coffers of large drug companies. In Rock's field trials in Puerto Rico, they said, he had exploited Third World women, using them as guinea pigs for an unproven and potentially dangerous drug.

There was some basis in fact for these criticisms. Early formulations used relatively high concentrations of hormones, which increased the risk of side effects and later health hazards. And it is true that both the risks and burdens of contraception fall almost entirely on women. And, yes, some of the clinical trials might be considered inappropriate or even unethical by today's standards. But in a sense the Pill is a victim of the very revolution in consciousness it helped bring about. If early formulations were not as safe as they could have been, it was more the result of ignorance than neglect. The side effects did not become apparent until large numbers of women had used the Pill. And the notion of what is proper and ethical in clinical trials of new drugs has changed drastically in the past 25 years; certainly the premarket testing of the Pill was no less ethical than the prevailing standard of the day. As for the suggestion that male doctors had no desire to find new and effective contraceptives for men, it's simply not true. Rock himself once devised an underwear liner for men that would keep testicles warm (sperm is only produced if the temperature within the testicles is about 97 degrees Fahrenheit). It was nicknamed the Rockstrap and for obvious reasons never enjoyed the popularity of the Pill.

Today's versions of the Pill are much safer than their predecessors, because doctors have learned that much smaller doses of the hormones they contain will do the job. And Pill boosters point to subsequent studies showing that the Pill creates virtually no additional risk of serious side effects when used by women who do not have such high-risk factors as smoking or diabetes; there are, in fact, some *beneficial* side effects, as outlined below. But even so, the Pill—indeed, contraception itself—remains a controversial subject. *Our Bodies, Ourselves,* published by the Boston Women's Health Book Collective, warns its readers that "if you take the Pill for many years at a time, you are in a sense part of a huge experiment" on its long-term effects. True enough, perhaps, but equally true of virtually any drug on the market.

As late as 1985, the American College of Obstetrics and Gynecology learned that contraception itself was still a touchy topic; all three major television networks rejected a public-service advertisement by the College designed to combat the rising tide of teen pregnancies. The spot, which said in part that "unintended pregnancies have risks—greater risks than any of today's contraceptives," was too controversial, the networks said. CBS, citing "network standards," said it rejected the spot specifically "because of the use of the word 'contraceptives.'"

On that low note, we'll leave the social history of you-know-whats and proceed to safer ground, a discussion of how they work.

Where Babies Come From

A baby, it's said, begins as a gleam in his father's eye—an apt description, perhaps, but not a particularly accurate one from a physiological point of view. The long journey toward birth actually begins in the hypothalamus, a tiny structure that lies just at the base of the brain. The hypothalamus plays a role in regulating many bodily processes, including reproduction. In women, it starts the process of ovulation—that is, production

of an egg capable of fertilization—by release of a special substance called *gonadotropin-releasing hormone,* or GnRH for
short.

Hormones, including GnRH, are chemicals produced by
certain glands and carried by the bloodstream to other organs,
where they stimulate a particular bodily process to occur. In
the case of GnRH, it doesn't have far to travel, for it acts on the
pituitary gland, which lies just below the hypothalamus. Once
there, it stimulates the pituitary gland to produce two
gonadotropins (hence the name) known as *follicle-stimulating
hormone* (FSH) and *luteinizing hormone* (LH).

The next stop on the hormone relay are the ovaries themselves. Here FSH and LH encounter *ova*—unfertilized eggs—
that wait in a kind of suspended animation. Each is surrounded
by a cluster of cells known as a *follicle,* and when FSH and LH
arrive on their monthly rounds to one or the other ovary (the
ovaries usually take turns releasing eggs), they set off a mad
race among several follicles to be the first to develop and
release a mature egg. Ordinarily, there's only one winner to this
race, for once a follicle is mature, it begins secreting its own
hormones, which shut down competing follicles.

As the ovum within matures, this follicle grows larger and
larger, until it bursts and releases the ovum from the ovary. But
its work is not done yet. It becomes transformed into a structure called the *corpus luteum* (Latin for "yellow body," and so
named because it takes on a yellow hue), which begins to
secrete additional hormones, including *progesterone*. These
hormones prepare the reproductive organs to receive and nurture a fertilized egg. If the egg that was released is fertilized by
a sperm cell, it sends a chemical message back home to the
follicle-turned-corpus-luteum, which then continues to secrete
hormones. If the ovum isn't heard from, the corpus luteum
fades away after about two weeks.

How the Pill Prevents Pregnancy

As the follicle (and later, the corpus luteum) mature, they
produce two important hormones, estrogen and progesterone.
When pregnancy occurs, the continued production of these
two hormones supports the development of the *endometrium*—
the soft lining of the uterus that nurtures the developing em-
bryo. The high levels of estrogen circulating in the bloodstream

also prevent the pituitary gland from producing FSH, and thus prevent additional eggs from maturing for the duration of the pregnancy.

The Pill contains estrogen and progestin (a synthetic form of progesterone); the estrogen, in effect, fools the pituitary into thinking that pregnancy has occurred, with the ultimate effect being that no new ova are released. The progestin provides two backup effects: it thickens the plug of mucus at the entrance to the uterus, making it difficult for sperm to reach the egg, and it alters the endometrium in such a way that even if an egg is fertilized, it cannot implant itself and begin to develop.

A woman takes a pill a day for three weeks out of a four-week cycle (many packages include a week's worth of dummy pills just to make it easier to remember to take them); after the last one, the sudden drop in estrogen and progesterone levels bring on menstruation. The following month, the cycle begins again.

Making the Pill Safer

Because most of the adverse effects of birth control pills are linked to estrogen (see below), newer preparations contain only one fifth to one half as much estrogen as earlier versions. Lower estrogen levels do, however, increase the likelihood of irregular menstrual periods and breakthrough bleeding (that is, bleeding during the middle of the menstrual cycle), and so it's sometimes necessary for a doctor to adjust the dosage before the right one is found.

There is, in addition, a newer type of birth control pill, the "minipill," that contains no estrogen at all. Minipills rely on progestin's effects alone, and thus aren't quite as effective as traditional, or "combination," pills. Also, like low-estrogen pills, they can cause missed or irregular periods and breakthrough bleeding, drawbacks that have discouraged their widespread use.

Problems with the Pill

While much of the early furor over the Pill concerned its effects on morality, a second wave of criticism—much of it from formerly enthusiastic supporters—involved the hazards it posed for women who were taking it. In 1969 a book by Bar-

bara Seaman called *The Doctor's Case Against the Pill* first
brought to the public eye some of the hazards associated with
oral contraceptives. Since that time, the seriousness of these
hazards has continued to be the subject of heated debate.

The following facts, at least, are clear. The Pill does create
a risk of possibly fatal blood clots, high blood pressure, loss of
fertility, heart attacks, and mostly benign liver tumors. It may
also be linked to gallbladder disease, although the evidence
isn't clear. For women who are older than 35, the risk of blood
clots and heart disease is increased significantly; smoking also
increases the risk of cardiovascular disease tremendously.
Women older than 35 who take the Pill and smoke heavily are
39 times as likely to suffer from cardiovascular disease as
women who neither smoke nor use the Pill. But for women
younger than 35 who do not smoke, the overall health risks are
much less—especially with low-estrogen preparations.

In addition, the Pill does have some secondary health
benefits. Women taking the Pill have a significantly lower incidence of benign breast changes, certain types of cancer and
anemia, premenstrual syndrome, painful menstruation, rheumatoid arthritis, acne, and pelvic inflammatory disease.

Does all this mean that the Pill is safe? The answer is,
unfortunately, a relative one, and in the final analysis each user
must weigh the risks and benefits for herself. Those who favor
the Pill are quick to point out that its health risks are much less
than either a pregnancy or abortion. That argument is a bit of a
red herring, however, for there are other forms of birth control
that have no discernible health risks. But they, in turn, are less
convenient and generally less effective than the Pill, so ultimately the question is one of whether convenience and protection are worth the risk. For whatever reasons, more than 10
million American women have apparently decided that they
are, and today the Pill is the most widely used reversible
contraceptive method in the United States and in the world.

Fertility Drugs

Fertility drugs, not surprisingly, are basically contraceptives in reverse. While the Pill contains estrogen, for
instance, the fertility drug *clomiphene* is an estrogen *antag-
onist*—that is, a drug that blocks the effects of estrogen. *Bromocriptine*, another fertility drug, works by reducing levels of

prolactin, a hormone that inhibits fertility. Ironically, early tests showed clomiphene to be a powerful contraceptive, equally effective in males and females—male and female rats, that is. In rats, small doses shut down the production of sex hormones in the pituitary gland and in females, reduced the size of the ovaries. In humans, however, it has virtually opposite effects, enlarging the ovaries and reversing infertility caused by naturally high levels of estrogen. Since its introduction in 1962, clomiphene has proved to be one of the mainstays of infertility treatment, and today it's successful in more than half of all cases of estrogen-induced infertility.

For women who do not ovulate because of a malfunctioning hypothalamus or pituitary gland, ovulation can be stimulated by a hormone known as *human menopausal gonadotropin* (HMG). A related hormone, *human chorionic gonadotropin* (HCG), mimics LH within the body, and is useful when infertility is due to low levels of LH.

Other hormones are sometimes useful in specific cases. Where infertility is caused by endometriosis or poor cervical mucus, doctors may even use estrogen and progestin—the same hormones that make up the Pill—giving these two drugs the curious distinction of promoting the same condition they prevent.

Drawbacks

There are, unfortunately, problems with these fertility drugs. For one thing, they don't always work. Infertility may be caused by something other than hormonal imbalances. The most common cause, in fact, is scarring of the fallopian tubes, which physically prevents the sperm and egg from coming together. In these cases, there are sophisticated new surgical techniques available, such as in vitro fertilization (IVF). "In vitro" is a Latin term meaning "in glass," and IVF is precisely that—fertilization that takes place not within the womb but in a glass laboratory dish under the watchful eye of a physician or laboratory technician. After the egg is fertilized, it's returned to the mother's womb, where it can be expected to grow and develop normally. Babies conceived by IVF are often dubbed "test-tube babies" by the press (a term borrowed from science fiction stories), but in actuality they spend only a tiny fraction of their existence outside the womb (and none of it in a test tube, by the way) and are in all respects perfectly normal infants. A true "test-tube baby"—that is, one that develops entirely outside the body—is far beyond the reach of modern medicine.

Even when such sophisticated techniques are employed, the treatment of infertility is still an inexact science, and neither drugs nor surgery can always assure a successful pregnancy. But that's not the only problem, for when fertility drugs do work, they are sometimes *too* successful. Unfortunately, it's easy to overstimulate the ovary and release too many eggs at one time, and a couple that arrives at the hospital in a two-seat sports car may need a small bus by the time all the dust has settled. Between 10 and 20 percent of all women who conceive with the help of HMG, for example, can expect twins; another 5 to 10 percent will find themselves with something more than two handfuls. Multiple pregnancies also increase the risk of miscarriage; fortunately, however, these drugs do not cause birth defects.

Wonder Drugs that Weren't: DES

It was, in the words of one advertisement, a "charm against abortion," and was prescribed to countless pregnant women in the 1940s and '50s to prevent miscarriages. Diethylstilbestrol (DES) is a powerful synthetic hormone and was known to cause cancer in animals, but physicians prescribing it to their pregnant patients had no idea that it could harm the developing fetus. In fact, the conventional wisdom 40 years ago was that the placenta formed a natural barrier that prevented most drugs from crossing over from the mother's bloodstream into the developing baby's. We now know that notion to be false; in fact, most substances in the mother's blood can traverse the placenta and affect the fetus.

Even after the myth of the protective placenta was discredited, nobody thought that DES had caused any problems. After all, millions of children had been born to DES mothers, and no apparent health problems could be traced to the drug.

That is, not until they became teenagers.

In the late 1960s, Dr. A. L. Herbst and his colleagues found eight cases of vaginal cancer in teenage girls seen at a Boston clinic. Until then, this type of cancer was exceedingly rare, and a gynecologist was likely to see few, if any, cases in a lifetime of practice. Thus, it was clear to Dr. Herbst that something was amiss.

The girls and their families were interviewed extensively as investigators sought to uncover the common thread. They considered just about every factor they could think of—up to and including household pets. In the end, they linked the cases to just three factors: bleeding during the mother's pregnancy, previous abortions or miscarriages by the mother, and the use of DES by the mother during the pregnancy. The association was strongest for DES; in addition, the link to DES was thought to be responsible for the relationship with the other two factors, since these had been just the sort of indications for which doctors had prescribed DES.

Based on their findings, Herbst and his colleagues concluded that DES was responsible for the cancer they'd seen in the eight girls. He began to collect information on other cases of vaginal cancer and within a few years had collected information on 91 other cases occurring in girls aged 8 to 25. In 66 of these cases, he was able to obtain information about drugs used by the mother during the pregnancy; of these 66, 49 reported having taken DES. The evidence was conclusive; potentially millions of DES daughters were at risk of developing vaginal cancer.

Ironically, DES didn't even prevent miscarriages; later research showed that the studies "proving" its effectiveness were poorly designed and poorly documented. In fact, evidence suggested that DES actually *increased* the risk of miscarriage. Thus, bad science, coupled with the myth of the protective placenta, had needlessly exposed a generation of girls to the risk of cancer.

What About Men?

Of course, successful ovulation is only half of the fertility equation. For a variety of reasons, sperm production may be impaired or absent in the male partner, and this is responsible in whole or in part for just about half of all infertility cases. A variety of factors can interfere with sperm production—everything from mumps to marijuana—but hormonal imbalances are only rarely to blame.

About a third of all infertile males suffer from varicocele, a condition similar to varicose veins in which blood pools in the veins surrounding the testicles. The pooled blood apparently raises the temperature of the testicles—acting as a sort of natural Rockstrap—and causes sperm production to cease. A relatively simple operation restores fertility in about 50 percent of these cases. The use of certain drugs—marijuana and alcohol, for example—may also inhibit sperm production, and initial treatment may consist of nothing more than abstinence. Where sperm production is low but not absent altogether, artificial insemination—that is, collection of the male partner's semen and placement of it at the entrance to the womb via a needle and syringe—may result in pregnancy. If the sperm count is too low, semen from an anonymous donor may be an acceptable alternative for some couples.

Among all these types of therapy, drugs play only a minor role. In the few cases where male infertility is caused by low gonadotropin levels, HCG and other hormones may help. Some doctors use clomiphene to treat infertile males for whom no underlying cause can be discovered, but the practice is questionable.

Fertility and Contraception: Looking to the Future

It's not clear what the future holds in the way of controlling reproduction. Concerns over the safety of the Pill have led to searches for safer preparations, such as the minipill. An increasing awareness of the fact that women bear an unfair share of the risks and responsibilities of contraception has sparked interest in developing effective, safe, and convenient male contraceptives. And the possibility of contraceptives that can be taken once a month or once a year has long tantalized researchers; injectable progestin is one candidate for such a long-term contraceptive, but undesirable side effects have thwarted the effort so far. As regards fertility, we can expect coming breakthroughs to involve surgery more than drugs, as doctors refine in vitro fertilization and related techniques. But whatever the future holds, we can be sure that the technical problems will be nothing compared to the social and cultural ones that accompany them.

9

Miracles and the Marketplace: The Story of Cyclosporine

There are undreamed-of wonder drugs all around us—cures, perhaps, for everything from upset stomachs to aging itself— lurking in the soil, in the air and water, gathering dust on some unknown chemist's shelf, even within our own bodies. Time and again in the preceding chapters we've seen examples of drugs that were beneath our noses but for one reason or another were undiscovered, unappreciated, misused, or misunderstood. Digitalis had been used as a folk remedy, probably for centuries, before it was introduced to science. Acetaminophen was discovered and then put aside for decades as an uninteresting and useless chemical compound. Calcium-channel blockers were little-known and seldom-used drugs for nearly 20 years before they were found to possess lifesaving properties.

All of this points to the fact that there is more than pharmacology and biochemistry to consider in any discussion of wonder drugs. There are also economics, politics, and marketing—that is, how a wonder drug makes its way from discovery to the drug store. In this chapter we'll do just that, using one of the most fascinating new drugs in all of medicine as a case study: cyclosporine. Its history is in some ways unique, and in some ways typical, of modern wonder drugs, and offers a fascinating glimpse behind the scenes of the multibillion-dollar world of today's drug industry.

Here then, is the story of the miracle called cyclosporine.

The Ancient Dream of Transplantation

Our account begins not in the laboratories of modern pharmaceutical houses, but three centuries after Christ in Rome, where lived the twin saints Cosmas and Damian. Cosmas was a physician and Damian a surgeon, and they are still remembered for their dedication to the healing of the sick.

Many legends surround the lives of these twin brothers, but the most remarkable one is the miracle of the black leg. The story is told that they had to amputate the gangrenous leg of an elderly church sexton. While the patient slept, the brothers replaced the diseased leg with one from an Ethiopian Moor who'd recently died. In the morning the old sexton awoke to find himself with two healthy legs, one white and one black.

Myth or fact? Either way the tale has fascinated men for centuries. A fifteenth-century German altarpiece depicts the saints, with a host of angels acting as assistants, performing the historic operation while the aged patient slept.

The idea of swapping body parts did not originate with Cosmas and Damian; it crops up again and again in ancient and modern myths. In ancient mythology there lived a creature called a chimera with the head of a lion, the body of a goat, and the tail of a serpent. In more recent times a book appeared, the title of which has since passed into common usage: Frankenstein, the tale of a man put together like a jigsaw puzzle from the body parts of corpses.

But the dream remained beyond the reach of medicine, seemingly forever. Following the discovery of blood types in 1900, it became possible to "transplant" blood, but more ambitious experiments showed that transplanting entire organs was a far more challenging problem. In 1902 a Viennese surgeon, Dr. E. Ullman, transplanted a kidney from one dog to another, and from a dog to a goat—all without success. French physician Mathieu Jaboulay attached kidneys from a dog and goat to the arms of two human patients; the organs worked for an hour. In 1936 a Soviet physician, Dr. U. Voronoy, attempted the first human kidney transplant; the kidney survived two days and even produced some urine, but then the patient died.

And then, on June 17, 1950, a historic event, rivaling the ancient feat of Sts. Cosmas and Damian, took place at the Little

168

Company of Mary Hospital in Evergreen Park, Illinois. Dr. Richard Lawler replaced the left kidney of Mrs. Howard Tucker, a 44-year-old woman in the last terrible stages of kidney failure, with the kidney of a woman who had just died of cirrhosis of the liver. Mrs. Tucker lived for almost five years after the operation.

But try as they might, other surgeons couldn't duplicate this success. In the flurry of transplant attempts that followed, most patients died immediately; only one lived for a few months. A French youth who lost his only kidney in an accident received his mother's kidney, which doctors hoped would be more compatible than a stranger's. It seemed to be, but only slightly so; the boy died after three weeks.

Two years later, surgeons at Boston's Peter Bent Brigham Hospital were successful when they transplanted a man's kidney into his identical twin, who was dying of kidney disease. The recipient recovered, married his nurse, and became a father. He survived for eight years. Surgeons at Peter Bent Brigham went on to perform 22 successful kidney transplants between identical and fraternal twins, but the larger problem of transplants between less closely related persons remained.

Although they still lacked the means to prevent rejection, all of this experience had at least given doctors a clear picture of why it occurred. It was, they knew, simply a case of the body attempting to protect itself.

One of the secrets to the success of the body's immune system is its versatility; it possesses the remarkable ability to respond to virtually any type of invading threat, no matter whether the invaders are viruses, bacteria, or other foreign material such as a transplanted organ.

This flexibility gives us protection against an almost infinite variety of pathogens—even ones we've never encountered before. That's an important feature from an evolutionary standpoint, since pathogens' rapid reproductive cycles give them the ability to mutate quickly into new and virulent forms. Humans mutate much more slowly, so the only long-term survival strategy is to have just this sort of all-purpose generic defense system as a guarantee against obsolescence.

For hundreds of millions of years, it has worked to our advantage. But in the case of transplants, it is the immune system itself that poses the most formidable obstacle.

The problem is that the recipient's immune system almost

invariably identifies the donated organ as foreign—and to the immune system, foreign means invader. The problem is similar to, but vastly more complicated than, that of blood transfusions. Transfusion of blood requires matching of only three blood antigens, but transplantation involves these three plus four major body-tissue antigens and a host of lesser, but still significant, antigens too. With so many variables, it becomes apparent why transplants usually only worked between identical twins.

Fortunately, the doctors didn't give up. If perfect matches were impossible, they reasoned, perhaps it might be possible to come at the problem from another direction. Attention focused on *6-mercaptopurine* (6-MP), a recently developed drug that was used to treat leukemia. 6-MP, it was found, had the ability to shut down the immune system for weeks at a time. In Britain, surgeon Roy Calne used 6-MP to perform successful kidney transplants in dogs for the first time. A derivative, azathioprine, was soon developed, which proved to be more successful and less toxic than 6-MP.

Azathioprine and other *cytotoxic* drugs used for immunosuppression work by killing off cells that are actively reproducing. Cells that are reproducing quickly, such as cancer cells or lymphocytes battling an invading organism, are more susceptible to the drugs than other body cells.

But azathioprine alone wasn't powerful enough to prevent rejection in most patients. In Colorado, Dr. Thomas Starzl looked into the possibility of enhancing azathioprine's effects by combining it with *corticosteroids,* naturally occurring hormones that had been used since the 1930s to treat a variety of diseases. These remarkable substances—commonly called steroids—have a wide variety of effects on the human body; one of their most well-known uses, for instance, is in skin creams to reduce inflammation, rashes, and itching.

Closely related to steroids' antiinflammatory effects is their ability to suppress the immune system. As part of the normal immune response, white blood cells secrete a substance that both attracts other infection-fighting cells and keeps them at the site once they've arrived. Steroids disrupt this chemical signal, in effect countermanding the white blood cells' order to attack the invader.

This property turned out to be the key to making transplantation a reality, as the combination of steroids and azathioprine enabled doctors to suppress the attack on mismatched tissues. Dr. Starzl later added a third agent to the mixture, antilymphocyte globulin, which also inhibited the action of the white blood cells.

But the price for all of this was steep, for these immunosuppressants also greatly impaired the patient's defenses against infection. Transplantation was a precarious and often unsuccessful balancing act, with the dosage of drugs high enough to prevent rejection, but not so high as to wipe out the immune system entirely. The closer the immunologic match between donor and recipient, the less suppression would be necessary, but the limited and fragile supply of suitable organs often resulted in matches that fell far short of the ideal.

Thus, transplant patients walked a fine line between organ failure and infection. When signs of rejection appeared, doctors would increase the dose of immunosuppressants and try to fight off the inevitable rounds of pneumonia, yeast infections, and other infections with powerful drugs. Patients were often kept in isolation to reduce their exposure to pathogens, but even such controlled surroundings could not always prevent infections.

Typically, rejection episodes came in waves, as if the immune system were an army mounting offensive after offensive. With luck, each episode would be less severe than the one before, as the body learned to tolerate its unwelcome guest. Eventually, the episodes would become mild enough to permit reductions in the amount of drugs. The immune system would, ideally, recover most of its ability to fight off infection, and the patient could lead a relatively normal life although still dependent on regular doses of immunosuppressants.

Despite the drawbacks, doctors used this approach to achieve some dramatic successes. Kidney transplantation became an accepted mode of treatment, though it wasn't always successful. Kidneys are well suited to transplantation, for a number of reasons. First, they keep relatively well, so it's possible to transport a donor kidney over long distances. Also, the surgery itself is very straightforward. Most important is the availability of a backup mechanism—namely, dialysis. Although dialysis is far from ideal as a replacement for a natural kidney, it can keep patients alive for years. Thus, transplantation failures are not fatal; the patient is usually no worse off than if he or she had not undergone the transplant at all. And by the same token, doctors didn't have to court deadly infections in an attempt to preserve the kidney; if infection became a severe problem, they could always abandon attempts at immunosuppression and sacrifice the kidney to save the patient's life.

But the real test of a broader role for transplantation came on December 3, 1967, when South African physician Christiaan Barnard performed the first transplant of a human heart. Here there was no turning back; the fate of the patient and his new heart were inextricably linked. The cat-and-mouse game between infection and rejection was literally one of life and death—and despite sophisticated preventive efforts and massive doses of antibiotics, South African greengrocer Louis Washansky died just 18 days after receiving the first transplanted heart, a victim of pneumonia.

Nonetheless, Barnard tried again. His next patient was 54-year-old Philip Blaiberg, a dentist from Capetown. The donor was a 24-year-old black man who had died of a brain hemorrhage. This time he was successful. Dr. Blaiberg lived nearly 20 months of virtually normal existence with his new heart, and was well enough to drive a car, swim in the ocean, and even write a book, *Looking at My Heart*.

The world's interest in this obscure African surgeon and his unprecedented accomplishment soon reached massive proportions. The effect was no less extreme in the medical world, and before long heart transplant centers were springing up like fast-food franchises. At Maimonides Hospital in Brooklyn, Dr. Adrian Kantrowitz transplanted a heart into a 17-day-old baby. The baby lived less than 7 hours. At Stanford University in California, Dr. Norman Shumway—Barnard's mentor—gave a 54-year-old man a new heart; the patient lived 16 days. In an eerie replay of the earlier experience with kidney transplants, surgeons all over the world tried to duplicate Dr. Barnard's feat—all without success.

Finally, nearly 5 months later, Dr. Denton Cooley of Houston, Texas, broke the run of failures. Everett Thomas, a certified public accountant, lived for 204 days, undergoing not one but two transplants. But in spite of a few more successes (one patient who received a new heart at the Medical College of Virginia lived for another 6 years and 3 months), the statistics showed that in most cases, heart transplants just weren't working. The rejection problem, combined with the difficulty of obtaining donors who were sufficiently close matches to patients, seemed virtually insurmountable, and the early enthusiasm began to sour. One after another the heart transplant programs were abandoned; while 101 people had undergone heart transplants in 1968, only 17 received new hearts in 1971. By 1975, the only U.S. heart transplant program still in existence was Dr. Shumway's at Stanford. With careful attention to the rejection process, he and his co-workers were able to achieve one-year survival rates of 60 percent.

But Shumway's limited success was seen as an aberration. Indeed, by the end of the 1970s the entire idea of organ transplantation was on shaky ground. Only kidney transplants had become well accepted, and even they were only sometimes successful. It seemed as though history would record the high hopes of the early seventies as nothing more than signposts pointing to a medical dead end.

The Discovery of Cyclosporine

The scene now shifts to Switzerland and the laboratories of the pharmaceutical firm Sandoz Ltd. Sandoz, like most other drug companies, had not forgotten the lesson of Benjamin Duggar and the discovery of Aureomycin®, and following Duggar's lead, they asked traveling employees to bring back soil samples to the company headquarters in Basel. Just as Duggar and his team had done, microbiologists at Sandoz hunted through these soil samples on a multimillion-dollar scavenger hunt, searching among countless species of fungi, bacteria, and other microscopic inhabitants of the soil for leads to new drugs.

Late in 1969, they came across some new fungi in soil samples from Wisconsin and Norway. The fungi produced two unknown but potentially interesting substances. By fermenting the fungal samples in vats, the researchers produced a mixture containing these substances. At first, the mixture didn't even have a name—it was simply referred to in tests as "24–556." Laboratory tests showed that 24–556 was able to kill a few species of fungus, most of which were insignificant from a medical viewpoint.

Already, this early in the game, it seemed as though 24–556 was just another one of thousands of pharmaceutical blind alleys. But, as Louis Pasteur stated in one of his guiding maxims, "Chance favors the prepared mind." In this case the prepared mind belonged to microbiologist Jean Borel.

Borel and his colleagues noted that 24–556 had an unusually low toxicity in animal tests—a seemingly unimportant fact, in view of the limited pharmacologic effects it had thus far displayed. But Borel and the others had learned from thousands of observations that substances produced by microbes, such as 24–556, often had other qualities besides their antibiotic properties. Since the substance had proved nontoxic, they decided to continue testing it.

Some months later, in January 1972, Borel discovered that 24–556 did indeed have other interesting properties, namely, its effects on the immune system. Testing the substance in mice, he found that it suppressed the immune system, much like steroids or cytostatic drugs. But here was a surprise. Where other immunosuppressants killed white blood cells indiscriminately, this material seemed to spare them!

This was a remarkable find—if it was accurate. Unfortunately, two follow-up studies failed to bear out the initial experiment; 24–556 performed poorly as an immunosuppressant. But then two more experiments confirmed the results of the first. (Years later, Borel learned the reason for the failure of the second and third experiments; he had dissolved the drug in a different solvent to permit him to use more concentrated doses; other studies later revealed that mice absorbed this second solvent—and any drug dissolved in it—much more poorly than they did the first.)

By now Borel knew he was onto something. But changes at Sandoz very nearly scuttled the project. Senior management, it seemed, wanted to get out of the immunology business, and they decided to "integrate" the research in this area into other, more promising areas.

In his account of the discovery of cyclosporine, Borel describes the subsequent events in the dispassionate terms of a scientist and downplays his own evident skill at internal politicking: "This decision," he writes laconically, "much discouraged further progress with 24–556 and I had to insist in order to continue my earlier work." He reports with equal equanimity that the Sandoz management eventually came around, persuaded by the compound's powerful immunosuppressive qualities and its apparent lack of side effects.

By now, other scientists at Sandoz had succeeded in breaking down 24–556 into two components—27–400 (Cyclosporin A) and 27–401 (Cyclosporin B)—and Borel's work continued using pure cyclosporin A. (Later its official U.S. generic name would simply be cyclosporine.) He found that the more he learned about this substance, the more strange it seemed to be. Where other immunosuppressants had attacked the body's infection-fighting white blood cells indiscriminately, cyclosporine was much more selective in its action. It spared the infection-fighting cells while blocking the cells responsible for rejection of foreign bodies.

This was truly a remarkable discovery. Out of the blue, it seemed, an obscure fungus had appeared with the solution to a vexing problem of 20th-century medicine. Had cyclosporine been discovered just half a century earlier, it would have been discarded as utterly worthless. Even a decade or two earlier it probably would have been overlooked, since nobody screened new compounds for immunosuppressive activity in those days.

In fact, the entire story of cyclosporine's discovery has more improbable coincidences than a third-rate spy novel. What if Borel had used the second solvent in his first experiments, and thus failed to note the compound's immunosuppressive properties? What if senior management at Sandoz hadn't been persuaded to take a chance on this apparently unpromising line of research? The successful development of cyclosporine in the face of all these odds is itself a miracle of sorts.

Borel's experiments showed cyclosporine to be an entirely different kind of immunosuppressant, and one that promised to overcome the drawbacks of earlier drugs. By April 1976 the change of heart at Sandoz was complete; management upgraded development of cyclosporine to clinical phase A—full speed ahead.

At just about the same time, Borel unveiled his findings at a meeting of the British Society for Immunology. He presented data demonstrating the following points:

• Cyclosporine was the first *selective* immunosuppressant, inhibiting the cells responsible for rejection while leaving the rest of the immune system relatively intact.
• It suppressed chronic inflammatory reactions, but not acute ones, which meant that it could prevent rejection without impairing the body's ability to fight off infections.
• It inhibited the proliferation of white blood cells, but didn't kill them; thus, its effects were reversible.
• It was effective in all species in which it had been tested, including the mouse, rat, guinea pig, rabbit, and monkey (at this point, it hadn't been tried in humans). This finding offered encouraging evidence that it would have similar effects in man.

Borel's announcement was astounding, and it would prove to revolutionize the field of immunology. Almost immediately, researchers undertook animal studies to see if this amazing new substance could really live up to its reputation. Two British scientists, D. J. G. White and Roy Calne (the latter is the same surgeon who pioneered the use of azathioprine) undertook a series of animal studies, the results of which proved that cyclosporine was every bit as incredible as Borel had claimed.

Human Tests Begin

The next step was to see what happened when cyclosporine was given to humans. Almost immediately, though, researchers ran into a snag, for lab tests showed that the drug wasn't being absorbed into the bloodstream.

Borel, recalling the problems with the mice in his early experiments, guessed that the problem was in the way the drug was being given, that is, dissolved in gelatin capsules. He concocted a solution he thought would do the trick, a cocktail consisting of 500 milligrams of cyclosporine dissolved in a mixture of 95 percent grain alcohol, 3 percent Tween 80 (a nonionic detergent), and a little water. Borel himself volunteered for the test.

Again we have Borel's account of the historic moment, terse and to the point: "As a consequence, I got tipsy." But the experiment worked; lab tests showed the drug to be present in his blood in sufficiently high concentrations.

A minor problem with cyclosporine, incidentally, is the difficulty of finding a suitable solvent to ensure its absorption by the body. Today, patients take their cyclosporine dissolved in olive oil—less exhilarating than Borel's cocktail, perhaps, but certainly easier on the liver.

Clinical Trials Begin

The next step, clinical trials, is the most important and is one at which many promising new drugs vanish into oblivion. There are many things that can go wrong at this stage. The drug can fail to work as expected, patients may be unable to tolerate it, or it may work, but not nearly as well as animal studies suggested

But by far the worst that can happen is that the drug can

prove to have dangerous side effects. Although the first-stage limited testing in humans is designed to detect possible side effects, it provides only a crude guide to a drug's safety. The full picture cannot emerge until the drug is tested under actual clinical conditions on relatively large numbers of patients.

Sometimes, in fact, even these trials are not enough. For the past 20 years drug researchers have been painfully aware of the thalidomide tragedy in Europe, during which an estimated 8,000 children were born with birth defects caused by a drug so "safe" that it was available over the counter in West Germany (see p. 115). And yet despite additional precautions adopted after that experience, there have been other, similar instances: A heart drug called practolol was introduced in Great Britain in 1970; it caused hearing loss, permanent visual damage, and a variety of other serious side effects in at least 1,000 patients before it was withdrawn. A blood pressure medication called Selacryn®, introduced by the pharmaceutical firm SmithKline, sailed through clinical trials, but was withdrawn after reports of fatal liver damage began cropping up. (The Selacryn® affair also resulted in criminal charges against SmithKline, with allegations that the company had misrepresented the safety of the drug to officials at the FDA.)

These and other experiences underscore the hazards involved in giving new and unproven drugs to patients, even under the controlled conditions of a clinical trial. Nonetheless, many of the physicians who performed transplants were eager to try cyclosporine, encouraged by the results of animal studies and other early tests. In 1978, Dr. Calne began using the drug in kidney patients in England.

The trials did indeed reveal a new side effect: toxicity to the kidneys, which had not shown up before despite all the animal studies. Calne and his colleagues started with doses of 25 milligrams per kilogram of body weight and noted that six out of the original seven patients in the study suffered kidney failure. Assuming that the problem was caused by rejection, the researchers added other anti-rejection drugs to the regimen, but to no avail. After a few months of further study they concluded that the cyclosporine itself was to blame and reduced the dose to 10 milligrams per kilogram. But even at these lower doses kidney damage still occurred; in addition, the dose was too low to prevent rejection. Next they tried raising the dosage a little, but found that the two problems—rejection and kidney damage—still remained.

Even with all these problems, 8 out of the original 16 transplants worked—which meant that this new and unfamiliar drug scored about as well as the best conventional therapy in its first trial. But Calne and his colleagues weren't satisfied and looked for ways to prevent rejection and kidney damage. They did some detective work. Reviewing their patients' medical records, they found that long-term success seemed to be related to the promptness with which the new kidneys had begun producing urine after transplantation. The best cases had been those in which the doctors had used the powerful diuretic mannitol to promote urine formation at the time of transplantation. The researchers also concluded that using large doses of other immunosuppressants along with the cyclosporine did little good and might even be harmful.

Armed with these findings, they began using diuretics in their patients to promote urine production and waited for six hours after surgery to see whether the new kidney was producing sufficient quantities of urine. If all was well at that point, they used cyclosporine; if urine production was poor or absent, they used conventional treatment. If they did use cyclosporine, they reserved steroids and other "traditional" immunosuppressants for acute rejection episodes.

With these changes, the success rate improved dramatically. After a year, almost 80 percent of patients in the trial had functioning kidneys—compared with about 55 percent who received conventional therapy. Cyclosporine was clearly as spectacular in the real world as it had been in the laboratory.

More Side Effects—and the Specter of Cancer

The drug was not, however, entirely free from side effects. Besides the problem of kidney damage, Calne and others found that the drug could cause increased facial and body hair, gum disease, tremor, mild liver toxicity, and other relatively minor side effects. And as more and more researchers began conducting their own clinical trials, disturbing reports began to surface of an increased risk of lymphoma (lymphatic cancer). Calne encountered three cases of lymphoma among his initial series of 34 patients, and other researchers found instances of the disease as well.

The finding was not entirely unexpected, since it had occurred with other immunosuppressants. One theory held that the immune system destroyed developing cancers and that any drug that diminished the immune system would, of necessity, cause an increased incidence of cancer. Further research suggests that the truth is somewhat more complicated, but there remains an important link between the immune system and cancer. One current theory suggests that immunosuppressant-related lymphomas are caused by Epstein-Barr virus. The normally inactive virus becomes reactivated when the immune system is suppressed, the theory holds, and in turn promotes mutations in white blood cells. Whatever the reason for the formation of lymphomas, Calne and others found that the solution lay in lower doses of cyclosporine and steroids.

On to the United States

Based on these and other results, Sandoz obtained permission from the U.S. Food and Drug Administration (FDA) to begin making cyclosporine available for experimental use, and in 1979 clinical trials began at more than a dozen U.S. hospitals. For many of the pioneers in transplant surgery, cyclosporine provided the opportunity to pick up a line of research that had been idle for years. In Houston, Dr. Denton Cooley hadn't done a heart transplant in more than a decade; soon he would be doing more than one a month. In Pittsburgh, Dr. Thomas Starzl resumed his work with liver transplants, which thus far had had only a one-in-three chance of success. And at Stanford, where Dr. Norman Shumway and his colleagues had continued to perform heart transplants throughout the 1970s, doctors began preparing for an even more ambitious prospect, a combined heart-lung transplant.

Before cyclosporine, lung transplants were considered virtually impossible, because ordinary immunosuppressants interfered with healing of the connection between the new lung and the patient's windpipe. But in March 1981 Dr. Shumway and Dr. Bruce Reitz used cyclosporine to achieve a medical first. In a four-hour operation, they successfully transplanted a new heart and lungs into a 45-year-old newspaper executive, who recovered and eventually returned to work.

As news of these breakthroughs made headlines, it also created some misunderstandings. As far as the FDA was concerned, the drug was still experimental and therefore wasn't available to all transplant patients. The success of cyclosporine, combined with the obvious clinical need for an improved immunosuppressant, led the FDA to put the drug on the "fast track"—a special program that expedites the approval of much-needed drugs—but even so, the FDA would need a great deal of information on cyclosporine before approving it—information that could only be obtained by the slow and painstaking process of experimental trials.

Meanwhile, the evidence of cyclosporine's effectiveness and relative safety continued to mount. The ongoing studies showed that one-year survival rates for heart transplants rose from 59 percent to 81 percent. For kidney transplants, the drug increased the survival rate from 53–83 percent to 73–90 percent. The potential for kidney damage remained and required vigilance on the part of physicians who administered the drug. And lymphomas developed at a rate of about 5 cases in a thousand, but this was actually two to three times less than the rate seen with azathioprine, the immunosuppressant that was most commonly used in transplant surgery. The research also revealed that cyclosporine reduced the initial hospital stay for transplant patients by 30 to 50 percent and, by reducing the need for steroids, helped prevent such complications as brittle bones and ulcers.

The verdict was clear. Despite the side effects, cyclosporine was clearly the drug of choice for transplants. It had revitalized the entire field of transplant surgery and re-stored life and health to thousands of patients. In November 1983—after more than 10 years of laboratory study, 8 years of clinical trials, and experimental use in more than 5,000 transplant cases—the FDA approved cyclosporine for clinical use. In the words of Dr. Starzl, who had earlier praised the drug in testimony before the FDA, the availability of cyclosporine marked "the breakthrough we've been looking for—the key that unlocks the door to transplants."

Looking to the Future

The FDA approval of cyclosporine is not, of course, the end of the story. As the drug has gained acceptance as the drug of choice for transplants, a new problem has emerged—its high cost. Maintenance therapy with cyclosporine costs thousands of dollars a year, and for some patients, the cost itself becomes the major hardship. At hearings before the federal Task Force on Organ Transplantation, doctors told of patients who, because of the high cost of cyclosporine, had reduced their dosage without their physicians' knowledge—a practice that has sometimes resulted in rejection of the new organ. In addition, the high cost of the drug and the limited number of transplant patients made pharmacies reluctant to stock the drug, witnesses at the hearing said. Some, noting that kidney transplants save the federal government money by eliminating a patient's need for federally funded dialysis treatment, have suggested that the government should pay for cyclosporine prescriptions. Others, including the American Association of Retired Persons (AARP), have objected to this proposal; the AARP says that if the government pays for cyclosporine prescriptions, it should pay for other equally lifesaving drugs for senior citizens. In the meantime, chemists at Sandoz have been looking for ways to manufacture the drug less expensively—so far without success.

On the clinical front, cyclosporine may prove to be more useful than had previously been suspected. Researchers are now studying the drug's effectiveness against a variety of diseases, with particular emphasis on such autoimmune disorders as diabetes and multiple sclerosis, in which the body is attacked by its own immune system. One surprising finding was that cyclosporine is effective against malaria, and although its immunosuppressant effects make it unlikely that it will ever be used for this disease, this discovery raises the possibility that related compounds may someday be useful for treating quinine-resistant malaria cases.

One of the most intriguing areas of research with cyclosporine involves its use in cross-species transplants. Its immunosuppressive activity is so strong that for the first time ever, transplants between nonhumans and humans have become at least theoretically possible.

Perhaps the most startling indication of this possibility was the case of "Baby Fae," an infant who was kept alive for 20 days with the heart of a baboon. The Baby Fae case created a storm of controversy at the time; animal-rights activists condemned the taking of the donor baboon's life; ethicists pondered whether Baby Fae had been unfairly made the victim of a half-baked experiment; others questioned whether more conservative therapy, up to and including a human heart transplant, might have been possible.

But nearly lost in the din of all the accusations and counteraccusations was the promise that this historic event held for future victims of terminal heart disease. For the first time in medical history, a heart from an entirely different species was successfully transplanted into a human being and kept that human being alive for almost 3 weeks. And if that accomplishment can be improved upon sufficiently, if it ever becomes practical to replace worn-out or defective body parts with organs from chimpanzees, gorillas, and baboons, the implications are enormous—notwithstanding the objections of animal liberationists. With an abundant source of animal donors, no longer would doctors have to rely on organs harvested from some young victim of suicide or a tragic accident; no longer would infants need to die while their parents hoped for an organ that came too late or not at all; no longer would elderly patients be denied transplants simply because there weren't enough organs to go around. No longer would the miracle of transplantation be dependent upon another human being's death.

It is the hope for such a future that is the legacy of tiny Baby Fae—a hope that is kept alive by the miracle drug cyclosporine.

10

Everyday Wonders: Drugs for Common Ailments

Not all wonder drugs are as dramatic as penicillin or cyclosporine; many lead a much more low-key existence. They're close at hand, usually available without a prescription, and often taken on the recommendation of a friend or pharmacist rather than a physician. They don't save lives, perhaps, but they make life more livable for countless patients. Perhaps they should not be called "wonder" drugs at all, although it then becomes difficult to know just *what* to call them. Near-wonders? Minor miracles? For purposes of discussion, we've settled on the term "everyday wonders."

We've given these everyday wonders a chapter of their own for a number of reasons. First is the simple fact that it's hard to talk about them in the same breath as some of the major medical breakthroughs discussed earlier. A drug that reverses heart attacks, after all, is something altogether different than one that reverses baldness. Likewise, a drug that controls epilepsy is a lot more important than one for controlling migraine headaches. Each is useful in its own way, but to suggest that they are equally important would be a disservice to them all.

Why, then, include them in this book at all? The answer is simple: They *are* wonder drugs. If you look back to the list of characteristics we developed in Chapter 3, you'll find that the drugs in this chapter do indeed make the grade. They may not mean the difference between life and death, but they work. They improve our lives; they're safe and convenient. If you have any doubt that these are wonder drugs, simply ask any hayfever sufferer whether he would willingly surrender his antihistamines, or ask your doctor to tell you what cimetidine (Tagamet®) means to his ulcer patients.

Also, there's the undeniable fact that these drugs are *popular*—and that alone makes them worthy of our consideration. A recurrent theme throughout this book has been the profound and often overlooked effect that wonder drugs have had—not only on medicine, but on the very way we view our world. The fact that we can take a pill to dry up a runny nose may seem far removed from notions of man's relation to the universe, but perhaps there is a connection after all. Everyday wonder drugs give us a means of controlling the minor and not-so-minor bodily afflictions that we encounter in our daily lives. Is it too far-fetched to suggest that one side effect is a tendency to see illness and discomfort as problems to be solved rather than divine retribution or simply the lot of mankind?

Consider, for example, a subject that seems far removed from the world of drugs, the law. In recent years our legal system has been reeling under the effects of huge jury awards— far greater than any ever seen in history. A very large part of these awards are often for "pain and suffering" of an injured party.

Why do jurors come in with such huge awards for pain and suffering, and why now more than ever before? One factor seems to be that people today are less inclined to see pain and suffering as an inevitable part of the human condition; rather, they tend to see it as a "wrong" that demands compensation.

Can we, then, blame high jury awards (and, by extension, high insurance premiums) on everyday wonder drugs? Maybe; maybe not. But it is fair to say that by helping blunt commonplace ills, these drugs raise our expectations about life in general. And they raise our expectations about science, too, by fulfilling the promise it so often holds out: namely, that life can be a little easier, a little more enjoyable, and a little bit better than it was before.

Here, then, is a look at some of these everyday wonders. The list that follows is by no means exhaustive, but it does include many of the most effective and popular of these drugs as well as a few fascinating newcomers.

Drugs for Colds and Allergies

To judge by the displays of cold medicines seen in the typical drugstore, you'd think that all the resources of modern medicine have been brought to bear against some terrible scourge. But in truth modern medicine has little to offer the cold sufferer. None of these "medicines" actually cures a cold or even shortens its duration. For anyone hoping that doctors may someday concoct a real cure, there's more bad news. It's none too likely, at least not anytime soon. Colds are caused by viruses, so antibiotics have no effect on them. A vaccine is pretty much out of the question since there are a hundred or more different viruses that can cause a cold, and since the cold happens to be a disease for which immunity is short-lived.

Fortunately, our bodies do a good job of fighting off colds all on their own. About the best contribution that medicine can make is to make us more comfortable for the week or so it takes for a cold to run its course.

And despite all the brightly colored packaging, the slick commercials, and the oblique talk about "special ingredients," there are only a few basic drugs that are helpful in relieving cold symptoms, although there are other less effective (or even unproven) ingredients that find their way into cold preparations—mostly, it seems, so that manufacturers can claim that their product is different (and, by extension, better) than the competition.

Decongestants relieve stuffy noses and blocked sinuses by shrinking swollen blood vessels in the mucous membranes that line the respiratory tract. Drops or nasal sprays applied directly to these swollen membranes are the most effective, although they should be used sparingly to avoid a "rebound" effect—that is, increased congestion when you stop using them. *Phenylephrine* (the active ingredient of Neo-Synephrine® and other brands) and *oxymetazoline* (Afrin®) are two effective ones. If the drugstore's closed or you don't feel like going out, you can use ordinary salt water, which is a natural decongestant. (Dissolve a teaspoon or so of salt in a tumbler of lukewarm water; insert a dropperful or so in each nostril—*don't* try to use the whole tumblerful!) Salt water isn't as effective as some other decongestants; on the other hand, it doesn't cause a rebound effect.

Antihistamines are also used in cold medications, though it's questionable whether they actually do much good for colds. For *allergy* sufferers, on the other hand, they relieve runny noses, watery eyes, itching, and other symptoms. Most also tend to make you drowsy, although a new one, terfenadine (Seldane®), is claimed not to cause drowsiness. These drugs work by blocking the action of *histamines*—natural substances released by the body's cells as part of an allergic reaction.

Although allergy symptoms and cold symptoms seem similar, they occur via different mechanisms, which is why antihistamines don't usually work too well when you have a cold. They do, however, tend to dry secretions somewhat, and the fact that they make you drowsy may help you sleep.

The third major class of ingredients in cold preparations are analgesics, including acetaminophen and plain old aspirin. These help reduce fever and ease some of the aches and pains (see Chapter 7).

For *coughs,* the most effective relief comes from the narcotic *codeine,* which acts on the cough center to block the cough reflex. (Yes, those television ads are true; there really *is* something called the cough center.) Codeine was widely used in cough medicines in years past, but since it shares with other narcotics the hazards of addiction and overdose, it's less popular today. *Dextromethorphan* is a nonnarcotic cough suppressant that works much like codeine. Home remedies, such as a mixture of honey and whiskey, may also be helpful.

But before you reach for any kind of cough syrup, think twice. Especially if the cough is a productive one—that is, if it's bringing up secretions. It's serving a useful function, and you may not be doing yourself any favor by suppressing it. In addition, a persistent cough—one lasting more than a week or two—may indicate more serious trouble and should prompt a visit to a doctor.

Allergy Medications

Traditionally, allergy symptoms have been controlled by decongestants and antihistamines (see above). In addition, allergists sometimes use *desensitization* for severe allergies; the process consists of exposing the body (typically via injections) to greater and greater doses of the allergy-causing substance. In this way the body eventually "learns" to tolerate the offending substance.

A relatively new class of decongestants for allergy sufferers are prescription nasal sprays containing steroids (brand names include Beconase®, Vancenase®, Decadron®, and Nasalide®). They rely on the ability of steroids to reduce inflammation and swelling, and since they're only applied to the nasal membranes, they're free of the side effects of oral steroids.

A major drawback of these drugs is the fact that they have to be used *before* the nose gets stuffy. For that reason, they're not very helpful for colds. But allergy sufferers can take them on a regular schedule during times when they're most susceptible to hay fever symptoms. Since they have a different mechanism of action than other decongestants, they're sometimes used to help overcome the rebound phenomenon.

Another new antiallergy drug is cromolyn (Nasalcrom®). It's sort of a turned-around antihistamine; rather than blocking histamine receptors, it actually prevents the release of histamine from cells. Like the steroid nasal sprays, it must be used before allergy symptoms arise.

Allergies can be more than simply troublesome; they can kill. In rare instances *anaphylactic shock* can result after exposure to a bee sting, medication, or other allergen. The effects can be swift and lethal; blood pressure drops precipitously and swelling of soft tissues in the throat may cause suffocation. *Epinephrine* works with lightning swiftness to counteract anaphylactic shock. By constricting blood vessels it raises blood pressure and reverses swelling. Epinephrine has saved many lives, but anaphylactic shock occurs so quickly that it's only useful if it's close at hand—in a hospital, for instance. (Epinephrine has another important use, incidentally. It's a powerful heart stimulant and is often used in resuscitation attempts to restart a heart that's stopped because of electrocution, drowning, or a heart attack.)

Asthma Drugs

Asthma is a constriction of the bronchi and trachea, the hollow tubes that carry air to the lungs. They're made up of involuntary muscle fibers, which can't be controlled by conscious will the way an arm or leg muscle can. In asthma sufferers these muscles spasm, restricting the lung's supply of air. The spasm may be triggered by any number of factors, including stress, cigarette smoke, and exercise.

Bronchodilators, the mainstay of asthma treatment, relax

these breathing passages. The most common type of bronchodilators are *adrenergic drugs,* which are essentially beta-blockers in reverse (see Chapter 5). They stimulate beta receptors in the bronchial muscles, relaxing these muscles and permitting free breathing. Earlier adrenergics, such as epinephrine, have a drawback. They also stimulate beta receptors within the heart and so can worsen some heart conditions. (By the same token, beta-blockers such as propranolol can't be used by asthmatics, since they can provoke an asthma attack.) Newer compounds of adrenergic drugs (isoproterenol, isoetharine, metaproterenol, terbutaline, and albuterol) are more selective; they work almost exclusively on bronchial tissue and leave the heart relatively unaffected.

These drugs may be administered in any of several ways. In emergencies, epinephrine is often injected to bring about immediate (but short-lived) relief. In less severe cases, other, longer-acting adrenergic drugs may be taken in capsules that are placed under the tongue to dissolve. Another way of administering the drugs is by means of a pressurized inhaler, which shoots a fine mist of the drug directly into the bronchial passages.

Another class of asthma drugs are the *xanthines,* including aminophylline, theophylline, and a few related compounds. They work at the cellular level to relax the bronchial muscles. They're effective for longer periods of time than the adrenergic drugs, but they're considerably more toxic. Thus, their use requires close supervision by a physician.

Corticosteroids are powerful antiasthmatic drugs, but their other effects on the body (such as reducing the effectiveness of the immune system) have made them a drug of last resort for chronic asthma. Recently developed steroid sprays (see above) act only on the bronchial muscles and don't get into the bloodstream in significant amounts; thus, they're potentially more useful than systemic steroids such as prednisone.

Drugs for the Digestive Tract

Perhaps it says something about our culture that the best-selling prescription drug in America throughout much of the late 1970s was *cimetidine (Tagamet®),* an antiulcer drug. Perhaps it also says something that it was eventually kicked out of the number-one spot by propranolol, a drug to treat and prevent heart attacks (see Chapter 5). These two drugs have something other than their celebrity status in common: They were both discovered by British chemist James Black.

Ulcers are caused by excess acid secretions, which in turn are caused by histamines. Cimetidine is nothing more than an antihistamine for the stomach. Big deal, you say? In fact, it *is,* for ordinary antihistamines have no effect whatsoever on acid secretion. It took Black and his colleagues 10 years of looking at more than 10,000 compounds to come up with cimetidine, and on more than one occasion the program looked so unpromising that it was nearly shut down by its sponsor, the pharmaceutical firm SmithKline. Finally, though, in 1972, the researchers were ready to announce that they had discovered an effective new ulcer medication.

Just about everyone—including officials at SmithKline—was unprepared for the enthusiastic response that greeted Tagamet®. This, it seemed, was the drug the world had been waiting for. Sales soared, breaking record after record. By 1983, more than 30 million people around the world had taken Tagamet®, and sales had amounted to more than $800 million—almost twice as much as those of the previous number-one drug, diazepam (Valium®).

Despite its popularity and its proven track record for safety and effectiveness, cimetidine is not perfect. It tends to slow the absorption of other drugs, and so dosages have to be adjusted accordingly. There's some concern over a cancer risk as well; by reducing the amount of acid present in the stomach, the drug permits the growth of bacteria, which in turn may produce elevated levels of carcinogenic chemicals called nitrosamines. It's too soon to tell whether this risk is theoretical or real, but some doctors recommend that cimetidine users take between 2,000 and 4,000 milligrams of vitamin C a day, since vitamin C has been shown to block the formation of nitrosamines.

There are a few other antiulcer medications available. Good old-fashioned *Maalox®* is about as good as cimetidine—though it's much less convenient, since you have to take a lot of it. A new drug that works much like cimetidine is *ranitidine* (Zantac®). It appears to be less likely to interact with other medications, and the incidence of side effects seems to be lower than for cimetidine. Yet another drug, *sucralfate* (Carafate®), works in a different fashion. It doesn't reduce stomach acid (hence, it doesn't promote the formation of nitrosamines);

Wonder Drugs That Weren't: Dinitrophenol

During the First World War, French munitions workers often developed a peculiar illness, marked by sweating, fever, weight loss, and other symptoms. The cause was the TNT with which they worked, which researchers had earlier shown to increase the metabolic rate of animals, sometimes to the point of death.

In 1931 a group of scientists at Stanford University sought to capitalize on the ability of dinitrophenol, a close chemical relative of TNT, to step up the metabolic rate. While recognizing that the chemical was toxic, even fatal, in large doses, they concluded that it could be used safely in smaller doses as an aid to weight loss. They did, however, caution that their discovery be used only under the supervision of a physician.

But this new, painless means of dieting soon became immensely popular, and the researchers' warnings were promptly ignored. Before long, it was available without prescription from 20 different drug companies, and was advertised as being "absolutely safe when taken in accordance with directions." Yet the drug was far from safe; toxic reactions involving the bone marrow, white blood cells, and the skin were soon being described in the medical literature; nine deaths were reported. Even with these findings, the drug remained popular, and as many as a million people were believed to have taken it to lose weight or simply cure a "low metabolism."

Then, in 1935, a new and unexpected side effect began to appear in the literature: cataracts. No one had ever observed cataracts in the animal studies, but soon it was clear that an epidemic was occurring among people using dinitrophenol. One observer estimated that approximately one user in 100 lost his or her sight; the damage was irreversible, although usually it could be corrected by surgery.

Across the world, dinitrophenol was banned outright or restricted to sale by prescription only. In the United States, however, the FDA was unable to act under the then-current drug laws. Many states passed laws making dinitrophenol a prescription drug, but only California prohibited its sale altogether. In 1938, the FDA received broader powers under the new Food, Drug, and Cosmetic Act and was at last able to remove dinitrophenol from the marketplace.

rather, it forms a sort of chemical Band-Aid® within the stomach, coating the ulcer and preventing the stomach acid from attacking it. Side effects and drug-interaction problems are virtually nonexistent, since sucralfate isn't absorbed into the body.

For less serious stomach ailments, ordinary *antacids* can often provide relief. They chemically interact with stomach acid to "buffer" it, that is, render it less acidic. They may be either systemic (that is, affecting the entire body) or nonsystemic; a major drawback of the systemic ones is that they contain a lot of sodium, which is bad for persons with congestive heart failure, high blood pressure, and other illnesses requiring a low-sodium diet. Other medications include *simethicone,* a chemical that breaks up gas bubbles; *Phosphorated carbohydrate solution (Emetrol®)* and *Compazine®* (a prescription medication related to Valium®), which help control nausea; and Dramamine® and scopolamine, which are effective for motion sickness.

Trouble Down South

Farther down the digestive tract lurk those twin nemeses, constipation and diarrhea.

Unlike the weather, nobody likes to talk about constipation, but a lot of people try to do something about it. At least that's what the evidence says. There are more than *seven hundred* different brands of laxatives on the market today. The simple fact is that of all these remedies, the best is almost always simple patience. Laxatives tend to be habit-forming and are seldom necessary. Lots of roughage in the diet helps keep the system in order, as do a regular routine, exercise, and a clean conscience (stress can lead to constipation). In some cases, constipation may be caused by certain drugs or foods, or very commonly by a disruption of established routines. In all these cases, everything usually straightens itself out in a few days. If it doesn't, a visit to the doctor is warranted to rule out more serious causes.

Like constipation, diarrhea is a symptom, not a disease, and while it can be inconvenient or even painful, it's usually not dangerous. This wasn't always so; one of the great killers of the last century, cholera, caused diarrhea so severely that the body's chemical balance was fatally disrupted. Victims often died within 24 hours of the first appearance of symptoms.

The underlying cause of diarrhea may be a flu virus, new intestinal microbes from unfamiliar food or water (travelers' diarrhea), proliferation of intestinal bacteria caused by antibiotics, or poisoning from food contaminated by salmonella or other bacteria.

Narcotics (for example, paregoric and Lomotil®) are the most effective antidiarrheal drugs available, but they require a prescription. Narcotics (see also Chapter 7) work against diarrhea by slowing peristalsis—the rhythmic contractions that move material through the digestive tract. By slowing the rate at which the material passes through the intestines, these drugs permit excessive water to be absorbed from the stools before they reach the rectum.

Kaolin/pectin mixtures (Kaopectate®, for example) are less effective than narcotics, but often they do work and they are readily available. Kaolin works by coating bacteria and the poisons they produce and transporting them through the digestive system, thereby removing the source of the diarrhea. Pectin is believed to have a similar effect, though it's not entirely clear how it works. Other over-the-counter drugs that work by similar mechanisms include activated charcoal and activated attapulgite.

One substance is a sort of switch-hitter, finding its way into both laxatives and antidiarrheal preparations: *polycarbophil*. It works like a sponge, absorbing excess water and swelling up in the process. The added bulk helps prevent constipation, while the water-absorbing properties help dry up loose or watery stools.

More Everyday Wonders:
Secrets of the Skin Trade

Oh, the things we do to our skin! In the name of beauty, we paint it, pluck it, pierce it,and tuck it. We lie on the beach until we burn it bright red, we try to make hair grow on it where it doesn't belong, and we remove hair from where it *does* belong. We perfume it and color it with rouge; we take pictures of it— often lots of it—to help sell whiskey, fast cars, stereos, and even drugs

Being on the cutting edge as it were, our skin picks up a lot of major and minor ailments all on its own. A stroll through the forest or a sinkful of dishes may leave us with a nasty rash; too much exposure to the sun may cause wrinkles, age spots, or even cancer. Bruises, bumps, scrapes, and cuts—no other organ is quite so abused just by the hazards of daily living.

Fortunately, there's effective relief, often available over the counter, for many of these injuries and insults. Following is a brief overview.

Contrary to popular mythology, *acne* isn't caused by diet or poor personal hygiene; it's caused by secretions from glands within the skin known as *sebaceous glands*. They produce an oily substance known as *sebum,* which reaches the surface of the skin via hair follicles. When sebum production is excessive—say, because of the hormonal changes that come about with adolescence—it can combine with dead skin cells to form a plug that blocks up the follicle. The sebum continues to build up behind the blockage, resulting in that painful scourge of prom queens, the common pimple. If the buildup is severe enough, tissue around the buildup can break down and infection can set in—in other words, a case of acne can develop.

Eventually, most people outgrow acne. But it may take as long as ten years before the victim's hormonal situation straightens itself out. In addition, there is the possibility of scarring, as well as the fact that acne is increasingly persisting well beyond adolescence. Oily cosmetics and oral contraceptives may be partly to blame for this, since the phenomenon mostly affects women.

For all these reasons—not to mention the emotional toll that acne can take—there's been a great deal of research over the years into this disease and potential treatments for it. The research has paid off in effective symptomatic treatment for even the worst cases.

For mild to moderate flare-ups, there are effective over-the-counter remedies that cause peeling of outer layers of skin. This action prevents the formation of plugs and so prevents buildup of sebum. Most also contain a water-alcohol base that helps dry out oily skin.

The most common of these keratolytic (literally, skin-dissolving) agents contain *sulfur, resorcinol, salicylic acid,* or *benzoyl peroxide;* of the four, benzoyl peroxide is the most potent. Incidentally, acne is one of the few skin conditions that is *improved* by exposure to the sun, since the sun's ultraviolet light increases the rate at which skin cells mature and slough off.

It's been found that in more severe cases of acne antibiotics can be helpful. They're applied as creams or ointments directly to the affected areas of the skin, a method that increases their effectiveness while minimizing such side effects as stomach upset, vaginal yeast infections, and allergic reactions.

Finally, for really tough cases, researchers have come up with a really tough drug: *isotretinoin (Accutane®)*. It's a relative of ordinary vitamin A, which has long been recognized as an effective antiacne agent. The only problem with using vitamin A itself is that it would require massive doses for long periods of time—so massive, in fact, that they would be toxic.

Isotretinoin is a man-made derivative of vitamin A, and it retains its antiacne properties while being considerably less toxic. It drastically cuts back on the amount of sebum produced, apparently by reducing the size of the sebaceous glands. In addition, it seems to act on the sloughed-off skin cells as well, though it's not understood just how.

In any event, the results are unequivocal. One trial found *complete* clearing of severe acne in 90 percent of patients who took it for four months. Even better, the results seem to be long-term or even permanent; some patients are reportedly free of acne three years after they stopped taking the drug.

However, there's something of a dark cloud around this silver lining. Although isotretinoin is much less toxic than vitamin A, it's not entirely free of side effects. Almost all patients taking the drug experience drying and chapping of the lips; about a third can expect dryness in the nose, mouth, and eyes. Other less common side effects include nosebleeds, muscle aches, hair loss, fatigue, and an increased sensitivity to sunlight.

Fortunately, these symptoms almost always go away after treatment stops, and they appear to be more of an inconvenience than a serious health hazard. More troubling is the fact that isotretinoin can cause birth defects if it's taken by a woman who's pregnant. Considering the high proportion of women of child-bearing age who might be candidates for isotretinoin, this is a serious drawback indeed.

Another drawback is the drug's expense. The full treatment, including visits to the doctor's office and lab tests, can cost as much as $1,000.

Because of the expense and potentially serious side effects, doctors reserve isotretinoin only for the most severe and resistant cases of acne. But in these cases costs and side effects are—in the minds of enthusiastic patients and their doctors, at least—outweighed by the prospect of overcoming this disfiguring and emotionally devastating disease.

Help for Other Skin Problems

So much for the teenagers; what does modern dermatology have in its bag of tricks for the rest of us?

For *rashes and itches* of all description, there are the drugs that are rapidly becoming as common and indispensable as aspirin: cortisone and related steroids. Poison ivy and the bites and stings of insects are actually allergic reactions, and *antihistamine creams* (for example, *Benadryl® cream* or *PBZ® cream*) are helpful for relieving their itch and inflammation. Oral antihistamines are also effective.

For *athlete's foot, jock itch,* and similar fungus infections, there are a variety of effective drugs. Mild cases are often treated with *tolnaftate* (Aftate®, Tinactin®) or with *undecylenic acid* (Desenex®, for example). If these drugs aren't strong enough, doctors have a number of more powerful prescription drugs, including clotrimazole, miconazole, amphotericin B, nystatin, and others. Where the infection involves nails, the beard, or the scalp, treatment is made more difficult by the fact that ointments and creams can't easily penetrate these areas and reach the offending fungi. Such cases can be treated with systemic antifungal drugs, either griseofulvin or ketoconazole.

Dandruff is caused by overachiever skin cells, which grow and slough off at such a rapid rate that they produce a noticeably flaky scalp. Antidandruff shampoos work by slowing down the rate of skin growth. The most popular and effective ingredients are *selenium sulfide* (found in Exsel®, Iosel 250®, Selsun®, and Selsun Blue®), *zinc pyrithione* (found in Danex®, Head and Shoulders®, and Zincon®), and *coal tar* (available generically and under many trade names).

The best kind of medicine for *sunburn* is prevention, but despite the warnings of dermatologists about premature aging of the skin and the increased risk of skin cancer from too much sun, we're not likely to see the beaches emptied anytime soon. After abstinence, the next best thing is moderation, which in most cases means the use of a good sunscreen. Sunscreens contain chemicals (the most popular being *para-aminobenzoic acid* and its derivatives) that absorb the sun's ultraviolet (UV) rays and so prevent them from being passed through to the skin. The UV rays are the bad guys as far as sunburn is concerned; visible light doesn't cause sunburn.

If the bad guys get through anyway (or, more likely, if you say what you say every year, namely, "I never burn"), a benzocaine-containing product (for example, Solarcaine®) might help ease the sting. Some authorities, however, feel that these preparations can actually be irritating to burned skin, and so recommend that you simply recite, "I promise to use a sunscreen next time, honest" for two or three days until the pain begins to subside.

Finally, there are two recent dermatologic "wonders" to treat that age-old human affliction, vanity. *Minoxidil (Loniten®)* was originally developed by researchers at the Upjohn Company as a blood pressure medication, but trials showed that it had the unusual side effect of unwanted hair growth. As blood pressure medications went, minoxidil was no star, but before long the scientists at Upjohn were rubbing minoxidil paste into the scalps of eager bald-headed volunteers. Results so far have been promising, and although minoxidil hasn't been approved by the FDA for treatment of baldness, the price of Upjohn stock rose dramatically on the strength of speculation that the drug could prove to be one of the biggest marketing bonanzas ever seen. Indeed, shiny heads across the country are already being slathered with homemade ointments made out of crushed-up minoxidil tablets—at a cost of a hundred dollars a month or more. So far, the stuff really does seem to reverse baldness, but the growth isn't always, shall we say, luxurious. Even worse (unless, of course, you own some of that Upjohn stock) is the fact that the new growth disappears once you stop using the drug.

And yes, there's something in Santa's bag for wrinkles, too: *Zyderm,* a highly purified form of beef collagen that can be injected into the skin to smooth out wrinkles. Collagen is a protein that occurs naturally in the human body, and it serves as a framework to support the skin and give it contours—much as rafters give shape and support to the roof of a house. Wrinkled skin is sort of like those old houses with sagging roofs caused by dry rot in the rafters; over time, the collagen frame-work beneath the skin begins to break down and the skin starts to droop. Zyderm fills in the defects and so presents an alter-native to facelifts or similar types of plastic surgery.

Because Zyderm comes from an animal source, there's the possibility of an allergic reaction, and so doctors must perform allergy tests before going ahead with the treatment. And like isotretinoin, the treatment is expensive—as much as $1200 for a complete facial overhaul. Also, the injected collagen tends to break down over time, and touch-ups may be needed within a year or so. All of these drawbacks may lead many to conclude that their wrinkles aren't so bad after all (that in itself is no small accomplishment), but Zyderm remains a useful and effec-tive treatment for many disfiguring conditions, such as scars from surgery, accidents, and severe acne.

Herpes

For a while, before we learned about AIDS, it looked as though herpes was going to be *the* most feared sexually trans-mitted disease of the eighties. It was even the subject of a made-for-TV movie, which starred soap opera heartthrob Anthony Geary as a sort of Albert-Schweitzer-among-the-lonelyhearts, waging a lonely antiherpes campaign at a swinging-singles re-sort. The network stressed the movie's public-information value (which says something about it as drama), and it was only one part of a veritable media barrage concerning the horrors of herpes.

Genital herpes can be a serious health threat, especially when the victim's immune system is undeveloped or poorly functioning. It can even be lethal to a newborn infant who is exposed to it during birth, and for that reason a cesarean delivery is necessary if the mother is suffering from or getting over an outbreak at the time of delivery. But the major impact of this viral infection, and the reason for all the media attention, is its stigma. It is incurable and easily transmitted by sexual contact, a combination that can create suspicion and anger in the bedroom. Persons with herpes often feel like sexual lepers, and it's not uncommon for blossoming relationships to wilt at the revelation that one partner has the disease.

Herpes is actually an entire class of viruses, various mem-bers of which cause such diverse diseases as chickenpox, mononucleosis, and cytomegalovirus infection, a flulike illness that sometimes results from blood transfusions. Two types of *herpes simplex* virus, type 1 and type 2, are responsible for cold sores and genital herpes, respectively.

There's no cure for herpes, though not for lack of trying. But *acyclovir* (Zovirax®), a drug introduced in 1982, does ease the severity of outbreaks. When the herpes virus is active, it secretes a chemical that combines with acyclovir to form an antiviral poison. Unfortunately, the herpes virus doesn't disappear entirely between outbreaks; it remains dormant in nerve cells near the spinal cord. When conditions are favorable—say, when the immune system is debilitated—the disease can re-emerge with a vengeance.

Acyclovir can lessen the severity of these recurrent attacks; if it's taken soon enough, it can even prevent them. Equally important, it can prevent the disease from being spread to others.

For many herpes sufferers, the drug provides little practical benefit, since the body's own immune system does a pretty good job of minimizing the number and severity of recurring attacks. But in those cases where the body's immune system isn't up to the job, acyclovir can be an important, even lifesaving, treatment.

In addition, research has shown that when acyclovir is given to people suffering from their *first* herpes attack, subsequent attacks are only about one sixth as frequent as in patients who received no treatment. Also, the fact that the drug seems to have very few side effects makes it possible for persons who suffer from frequent attacks to take it on a daily basis, and thus prevent flare-ups altogether.

Thus, although acyclovir isn't a cure, it is an important step forward in the treatment of herpes.

A Final Note: The Wonder Drug with the Heavenly Aroma

Before we leave this chapter, let's consider one last everyday wonder: coffee. For centuries, it's suffered from attempts to malign it, or even outlaw it. In the sixteenth century, Muslims outlawed coffee in parts of Europe, burning caches of the "irreligious" bean wherever they found it. The Christians, on the other hand, declared coffee an "infidel" beverage. Both religions later changed their minds.

Today, the coffee naysayers are as popular and as vocal as ever. Caffeine has been implicated, with varying degrees of success, in heart attacks, high blood pressure, anxiety, ulcers, benign breast lumps, birth defects, and even cancer. And yet, according to an article in *Hospital Pharmacy* by pharmacists Marsha A. Raebel and Jimmy Black, "the case against coffee is not clear." They note that 2⅓ billion pounds of the stuff is brewed in America every year, and eight out of ten adult Americans are coffee drinkers, consuming on an average 3½ cups a day. Caffeine, they say, is "the most widely used drug in Western society," and yet the many studies that have been performed concerning its effects are often contradictory and not always rigorously scientific. The more scientific studies have found that when caffeine is given to non–coffee drinkers, it does indeed have significant effects on heart rate, blood pressure, and other bodily functions. However, habitual caffeine users become tolerant to these effects, and there don't seem to be any long-term changes in the body resulting from chronic caffeine use.

On the positive side, caffeine can be a very important drug for management of premature infants, in whom it reduces the number of apneic (nonbreathing) spells. And it is an effective stimulant, and a far safer one than amphetamines. Even better, caffeine seems to be free of the many ill effects once ascribed to it. Careful scientific research has failed to find any link between caffeine and cancer, birth defects, or heart attacks. In fact, caffeine may actually *help* heart patients; a recent study of coffee-drinking heart patients showed that they were able to walk farther without heart pains after drinking caffeinated rather than decaffeinated coffee, and that their electrocardiograms were improved as well. In addition, it's virtually impossible to overdose on caffeine; it's estimated that you'd have to drink 80 cups of coffee to die from it, and we submit that 80 cups of just about *anything* would be lethal.

But our defense of coffee as a wonder drug transcends mere scientific evidence. It's more than a stimulant; it's an old friend and companion. It's a way to keep in touch with your co-workers at the coffee machine; it's an excuse to linger over the morning paper. And especially for those who labor with the printed word all day—the proofreaders, editors, and writers of the world—it is even more than all that; it is a way of life.

And that is why, in this chapter at least, coffee is the wonder drug to end all wonder drugs.

Appendix

Pharmaceutical All-Stars:
A (Somewhat Arbitrary) List
of Wonder Drugs

The list that follows shows some of the most safe and effective drugs available to doctors and patients today, cataloged according to the disease or condition they're used for. Like any such list, this one isn't all-inclusive, and we would expect other physicians to have favorites that aren't included here. Therefore, don't be alarmed if your doctor is giving you another drug for any of the conditions listed here; it may simply be the same drug masquerading under another name, a close chemical relative, or an alternative that your doctor chose based on his or her experience or because of your particular medical history. Also, note that the drugs are listed alphabetically under each entry; because each clinical situation is unique, we made no attempt to rank these drugs according to their effectiveness.

Here, then, are our nominations for the best drugs in medicine:

Allergies

Antihistamines   Cromolyn
Corticosteroid nasal sprays   Decongestants

Anemia (Pernicious)

Folic acid

Arthritis

Aspirin   Azathioprine
Auranofin   Ibuprofen

Asthma

Aminophylline
Corticosteroids
Epinephrine
Isoproterenol

Metaproterenol
Terbutaline
Theophylline

Cancer

Bleomycin
Cisplatin
Dactinomycin
Doxorubicin
Estrogen
Fluorouracil
Mclanoma vaccine
Mercaptopurine

Methotrexate
Monoclonal antibodies
Nitrogen mustards
Prednisone
Procarbazine
Thioguanine
Vinblastine
Vincristine

Contraception

The Pill

The Mini-Pill

Cough

Codeine

Dextromethorphan

Diabetes

Chlorpropamide

Insulin

Diarrhea

Kaolin-pectin

Drug Abuse

Alcohol:

Disulfiram

Cocaine:

Bromocriptine

Narcotics:

Clonidine
Naloxone
Naltrexone

Tobacco:

Nicorette®

Epilepsy

Carbamazepine	Phenytoin
Ethosuximide	Primidone
Phenobarbital	Valproic acid

Gallbladder Attacks

Chenodiol

Gout

Allopurinol	Probenecid

Heart and Cardiovascular Diseases

Beta-blockers	Nitroglycerin
Calcium-channel blockers	Procainamide
Captopril	Quinidine
Clofibrate	Streptokinase
Digoxin	Tissue-plasminogen activator
Lidocaine	

Hemorrhoids

Benzocaine	Pramoxine

Hypertension

Beta-blockers
Captopril
Clonidine and other antiadrenergic agents
Diuretics
Indapamide
Reserpine and other rauwolfia-derived drugs

Infections

Bacterial:	*Fungal (systemic):*
Aminoglycosides	Ketoconazole
Cephalosporins	*Viral:*
Erythromycin	
Penicillin	Acyclovir
Tetracycline	Amantadine
	Immune globulins
	Vaccines

Infertility

Bromocriptine
Clomiphene
Human chorionic gonadotropin
Human menopausal gonadotropin

Migraine Headaches

Ergotamine
Propranolol

Motion Sickness

Dimenhydrinate
Transdermal scopolamine

Myasthenia Gravis

Prednisone

Pain

Acetaminophen
Aspirin
Morphine and other opiates

Parkinson's Disease

Carbidopa-levodopa
Levodopa

Patent Ductus Arteriosus

Alprostadil
Indomethacin

Preterm Labor

Magnesium sulfate
Ritodrine
Terbutaline

Psychological Disorders

Anxiety and Insomnia:

Chloral hydrate

Diazepam and other benzodiazepines
Tryptophan

Depression:

Imipramine and other tricyclic antidepressants
MAO inhibitors

Mania:

Lithium

Schizophrenia:

Chlorpromazine and other phenothiazines
Haloperidol

Skin and Scalp Disorders

Acne:

Benzoyl peroxide
Isotretinoin

Dandruff:

Coal tar
Selenium sulfide
Zinc/Pyrithione

Fungal Infections:

Clotrimazole
Miconazole
Tioconazole
Tolnaftate

Itching and Inflammation:

Topical corticosteroids

Lice:

Lindane
Malathion
Pyrethrins

Wrinkles:

Collagen

Transplants

Antilymphocyte globulin
Azathioprine

Corticosteroids
Cyclosporine

Tuberculosis

Isoniazid

Rifampin

Ulcers

Cimetidine
Maalox®

Sucralfate

Sources

ACOG Gallup poll: "Americans Mistaken About Contraceptives." *American Medical News,* March 15, 1985, p. 16.

"ACOG Officials Criticize TV Networks' Rejection of Spots on Contraception." *American Medical News,* August 16, 1985, pp. 1, 25.

Altman, L. K. "Heart Attack: Rapid Change in Therapy." *The New York Times,* March 16, 1982, p. C3.

————. "New Therapy Appears Capable of Stopping Heart Attack's Progress." *The New York Times,* June 15, 1985, pp. C1, C2.

AMA Ad Hoc Panel on Pertussis Vaccine Injury. "Pertussis Vaccine Injury." *JAMA,* 1985, vol. 254, pp. 3083–84.

AMA Drug Evaluations, 5th ed. Chicago: The American Medical Association, 1983.

"An All-in-One Birth Control Pill, Abortifacient, Cushing's Treatment?" *Medical World News,* August 27, 1984, p. 51.

"Antihistamines Relieve Symptoms of Hay Fever Without Drowsiness." *Medical World News,* March 12, 1984, pp. 111–12.

Bisno, A. "The Rise and Fall of Rheumatic Fever." *JAMA,* 1985, vol. 254, pp. 538–41.

Bolotin, C. "Drug as Hero." *Science '85,* June 1985, pp. 68–71.

Bottcher, H. *Wonder Drugs.* J. B. Lippincott Co., 1964.

"Breast Cancer Vaccine Tested in Two Trials." *Medical World News,* June 13, 1983, pp. 10–11.

Busch, L. "Hearing Addresses Cyclosporine-Related Issues." *American Medical News,* June 7, 1985, p. 20.

Bylinsky, G. "Medicine's Next Marvel: The Memory Pill." *Fortune,* January 20, 1986, pp. 68–71.

————. "Science Scores a Cancer Breakthrough." *Fortune,* November 25, 1985, pp. 16–21.

"Calcium Channel Blockers Promising for Migraine, Cluster Headache." *Medical World News,* August 3, 1984, p. 21.

"Cardiac Pacemakers: Current Issues for Hospital Executives." *Issues in Health Care Technology,* March 1, 1985, p. 19.

"Cardioselective Beta Blocker Found Safe for Insulin-Treated Diabetics." *Medical World News,* June 7, 1982, pp. 148–50.

Chase, M. "To Doctor and Patient, Test of a New Drug is a Turbulent Experience." *The Wall Street Journal,* September 26, 1985, section 1, p. 20.

Check, W. A. "A Quantum Leap in Pharmaceuticals." *Medical World News,* January 1985, pp. 162–71.

———. "Epilepsy: New Tactics in an Age-Old Battle." *Medical World News,* April 23, 1984, pp. 51–73.

Clark, M., D. Witherspoon. "Heart Attack Damage Control." *Newsweek,* June 13, 1983, p. 52.

"Coffee Boosts Pain-Free Walking Time for Patients with Chronic Stable Angina." *Medical World News,* March 12, 1984, p. 137.

"Collagen Cited for Vocal Cord Repair." *Medical World News,* March 12, 1984, p. 20.

"Comeback for Heart Transplants." *Time,* August 23, 1983, p. 54.

Cooper, R., J. Stamler, A. Dyer, and D. Garside. "The Decline in Mortality from Coronary Heart Disease, U.S.A., 1968–1975." *Journal of Chronic Diseases,* 1978, vol. 31, pp. 709–20.

"Cosmas and Damian in the 20th century?" *New England Journal of Medicine,* July 30, 1981, p. 280.

"Countering Cancer Drug Resistance." *Medical World News,* July 22, 1985, p. 31.

Crudele, J. "Hair Growth Drug Seen as a Wonder for Upjohn." *The New York Times,* May 28, 1985, pp. D1, D11.

Cyan, E. D., L. Hessman. *Without Prescription.* New York: Simon and Schuster, 1972.

"Cyclosporine: A Mixed Blessing." *Medical World News,* March 25, 1985, p. 62.

"Cyclosporine: Primed for New Battle." *Medical World News,* July 8, 1985, p. 94.

"Cyclosporine Scores in Diabetes Trial." *Medical World News,* March 11, 1985, p. 111.

"Cyclosporine Therapy Results in Remission for 16 of 30 Diabetics." *Medical World News,* May 14, 1984, p. 67.

Dackis, C. A., M. S. Gold. "Bromocriptine as Treatment of Cocaine Abuse." *Lancet,* 1985, vol. i, pp. 1151–52.

"Does Aspirin Reduce Stroke Severity?" *Medical World News,* June 24, 1985, p. 8.

SOURCES

Drake, D. C. "Treating Cancer: A New Era of Excitement Begins." *Philadelphia Inquirer,* April 7, 1985, pp. A1, A16.

"Drug Eases Cigarette Craving." *Medical World News,* January 14, 1985, pp. 29–33.

"Drug That Can Revive Antibiotic's Knockout Power Now Being Marketed." *Medical World News,* September 10, 1984, pp. 26–27.

"Easing Cocaine Withdrawal." *Medical World News,* November 11, 1985, p. 128.

"European Cooperative Study Group for Streptokinase Treatment in Acute Myocardial Infarction." *New England Journal of Medicine,* 1979, vol. 301, pp. 797–802.

"First FDA-Approved Clinical Trial of Natural Body Opiate Begins." *Medical World News,* October 10, 1983, p. 7.

Gardner H. *The Shattered Mind: The Person After Brain Damage.* New York: Knopf, 1975.

Giannini, A. J., I. Extein, M. S. Gold, A. L. C. Pottash, and S. Castellani. "Clonidine in Mania." *Drug Development Research,* 1983, vol. 3, pp. 101–03.

Gold, M. S., C. A. Dackis. "New Insights and Treatments: Opiate Withdrawal and Cocaine Addiction." *Clinical Therapeutics,* 1984, vol. 7, pp. 6–21.

Gold, M. S., A. L. C. Pottash, H. D. Kleber, and I. Extein. "Opiate Withdrawal, Clonidine, and Serum PRL. Evidence Against a Dopamine Hypothesis." *Neuroendocrinology Letter,* 1980, vol. 2, pp. 351–56.

Gold, M. S., A. L. C. Pottash, H. D. Kleber, I. Extein, and W. J. Annitto. "Antinoradrenergic Medications, Lofexidene and Clonidine Reverse and Suppress Opiate Withdrawal in Man." In: C. Perris, G. Struwe, and B. Jansson, eds. *Biological Psychiatry,* 1981: Proceedings from the IIIrd World Congress of Biological Psychiatry. New York: Elsevier, 1981.

Gold, M. S., A. L. C. Pottash, D. R. Sweeney, I. Extein, and W. J. Annitto. "Lofexidene Blocks Acute Opiate Withdrawal." In: "Problems of Drug Dependence: Proceedings of the 43rd Annual Scientific Meeting." Research monograph series 41. Washington, D.C.: National Institute on Drug Abuse.

Gold, M. S., A. L. C. Pottash, D. R. Sweeney, I. Extein, and W. J. Annitto. "Opiate Detoxification with Lofexidene." *Drug and Alcohol Dependence,* 1981, vol. 8, pp. 307–15.

Gold, M. S., A. L. C. Pottash, D. R. Sweeney, and H. D. Kleber. "Efficacy of Clonidine in Opiate Withdrawal: A Study of Thirty Patients." *Drug and Alcohol Dependence,* 1980, vol. 6, pp. 201–08.

Gold, M. S., A. L. C. Pottash. "The Neurobiological Implications of Clonidine HCI." *Annals of the New York Academy of Sciences,* 1981, vol. 362, pp. 191–202.

Gold, M. S., A. L. C. Pottash, and I. Extein. "Clonidine in Acute Opiate Withdrawal." *New England Journal of Medicine,* 1980, vol. 302, pp. 1421–22.

Gold, M. S., A. L. C. Pottash, D. R. Sweeney, and H. D. Kleber. "Effect of Methadone Dosage on Clonidine Detoxification Efficacy." *American Journal of Psychiatry,* 1980, vol. 137, pp. 375–76.

Gold, M. S., A. L. C. Pottash, and H. D. Kleber. "Outpatient Clonidine Detoxification." *Lancet,* 1981, vol. i, p. 621.

Gold, M. S., A. L. C. Pottash, D. R. Sweeney, R. K. Davies, and H. D. Kleber. "Clonidine Decreases Opiate Withdrawal-Related Anxiety." *Substance and Alcohol Actions/Misuse,* 1980, vol. 1, pp. 239–46.

Gold, M. S., A. L. C. Pottash, D. R. Sweeney, and H. D. Kleber. "Opiate Withdrawal Using Clonidine: A Safe, Effective, and Rapid Nonopiate Treatment." *JAMA,* 1980, vol. 243, pp. 343–46.

Gold, M. S., A. L. C. Pottash. "Endorphins, Locus Coeruleus, Clonidine and Lofexidine: A Mechanism for Opiate Withdrawal and New Nonopiate Treatments." *Advances in Alcohol & Substance Abuse,* 1981, vol. 1, pp. 33–52.

Gold, M. S., A. L. C. Pottash. "Naloxone and Naltrexone: Endorphin Antihormones." In: M. K. Agarwal, ed. *Hormone Antagonists.* New York: Walter de Gruyter, 1982.

Gold, M. S., W. S. Rea. "The Role of Endorphins in Opiate Addiction, Opiate Withdrawal, and Recovery." *Psychiatric Clinics of North America,* 1983, vol. 6, pp. 489–520.

Goldman, L., E. F. Cook. "The Decline in Ischemic Heart Disease Mortality Rates." *Annals of Internal Medicine,* 1984, vol. 101, pp. 825–36.

Goodfield, J. "The Last Days of Smallpox." *Science '85,* October 1985, pp. 58–66.

Goodman, S., A. Gilman. *The Pharmacological Basis of Therapeutics,* 5th and 6th eds. New York: Macmillan, 1975, 1983.

Green, R. "Vaccine Development: On the Verge of a New

Era?" *Medical World News,* February 25, 1985, pp. 46–63.

Gruson, L. "Treatment of Stroke: Advances Bring New Hope." *The New York Times,* February 26, 1985, pp. C1, C5.

"Hair-Raising Drug." *Newsweek,* June 10, 1985, p. 72.

Hall, A. "The Race for Miracle Drugs." *Business Week,* July 22, 1985, pp. 92–97.

Hamilton, J. O., R. Rhein, Jr. "The Gene Doctors: Scientists Are on the Verge of Curing Life's Cruelest Diseases." *Business Week,* November 18, 1985, pp. 76–85.

Halberstam, M. "Living in the Coronary Culture." *Esquire,* May 1981, pp. 68–75.

Harkness, R. *OTC Handbook,* second edition. Oradell, NJ: Medical Economic Publishing Company, 1983.

Hecht, A. "Slashing Away at Red Tape in the Drug Approval Process." *FDA Consumer,* February 1983, pp. 10–11.

———. "Sulfa: Yesterday's Hero Is Still Taking Bows." *FDA Consumer,* October 1984, pp. 8–11.

———. "Prompt Drug Approvals, More Innovation Sought." *FDA Consumer,* September 1983, pp. 12–14.

"High Recurrence Prompts Questions About Efficacy of Anti-ulcer Therapy." *Medical World News,* September 26, 1983, p. 24.

Hoeg, J. M., R. E. Gregg, and H. B. Brewer, Jr. "An Approach to the Management of Hyperlipoproteinemia." *JAMA,* 1986, vol. 255, pp. 512–21.

"Hundreds Seek New Hair Growth." *Medical World News,* May 23, 1983, p. 35.

Ismach, J. M. "Man vs. Microbes: Grappling with Resistance." *Medical World News,* February 13, 1984, pp. 43–57.

"IV Streptokinase Works, but Can It Beat Plasminogen Activator?" *Medical World News,* June 25, 1984, pp. 8–9.

Keh, L., P. J. Menard. "The Use of Calcium Channel Blockers in Asthma and Hypertension." *Hospital Pharmacy,* 1984, vol. 19, pp. 419–21.

Kline, D. "The Anatomy of Addiction." *Equinox,* September/October 1985, pp. 77–86.

Klippel, J. H., J. L. Decker. "Methotrexate in Rheumatoid Arthritis." *New England Journal of Medicine,* 1985, vol. 312, pp. 853–54.

Kolata, G. B. "Drug Found to Help Heart Attack Survivors." *Science,* 1981, vol. 214, pp. 774–75.

————. "Drug Transforms Transplant Medicine." *Science,* July 1, 1983, pp. 40–42.

————. "New Heart Attack Treatment Discussed." *Science,* 1981, vol. 214, pp. 1229–30.

Larkin, T. "Cortisone: The Limits of a Miracle." *FDA Consumer,* September 1985, pp. 27–29.

Lee, G., D. T. Mason. "Percutaneous Transluminal Coronary Recanalization: A New Approach to Acute Myocardial Infarction Therapy with the Potential for Widespread Application." *American Heart Journal,* 1981, vol. 101, pp. 121–23.

Leonard, G. "Margaret Chesney's Affair of the Heart." *Esquire,* December 1984, pp. 74–82.

"Lessons from Ancient Ancestors: Potassium for Hypertension?" *Medical World News,* March 11, 1985, pp. 58–59.

Levine, A. " 'Gilding the Lily': A DES Update." *Trial,* December 1984, pp. 18–22.

Lieber, J. "Coping with Cocaine." *Atlantic,* January 1986, pp. 39–48.

"Manipulation of Immune System Succeeds in Fight Against Cancer." *Hospital Technology Series,* January 1986, p. 1.

Marcus, A. J. "Editorial Retrospective: Aspirin as an Antithrombotic Medication." *New England Journal of Medicine,* 1983, vol. 309, pp. 1515–17.

McIlrath, S. "Vaccine Issue Foremost in Clinical Medicine." *American Medical News,* January 4, 1985, p. 13.

Merz, B. "Good Genes Gone Bad: Closing in on the Oncogene Link with Cancer." *Medical World News,* April 8, 1985, pp. 89–107.

"Minoxidil: A Brief Boost to the Scalp." *Medical World News,* April 23, 1984, p. 34.

"Monoclonal Antibodies Fight Bacteria." *Hospitals,* January 16, 1985, p. 64.

"Monoclonal Antibodies Used as Aid to Fight Transplant Rejections." *Medical World News,* August 8, 1983, p. 66.

"Monoclonal Antibody Use Expands to Protect Against Endotoxic Shock." *Medical World News,* June 24, 1985, p. 36.

"Multidrug Hodgkin's Regimens Bring Up to 100% in Remission." *Medical World News,* January 9, 1984, p. 42.

Myers, J. A. *Captain of All These Men of Death.* St. Louis: W. H. Green, 1977.

"New Drug Aids Transplant Patients, Hurts Wallet." *St. Petersburg Times,* January 13, 1985, p. B2.

"New Technology: Percutaneous Transluminal Coronary Angioplasty." *Issues in Health Care Technology,* November 5, 1981, p. 2.

"New Technology: Streptokinase Thrombolysis of Coronary Arteries." *Issues in Health Care Technology,* September 5, 1982, p. 1.

"New Vaccines Show Potential of Fending Off Melanoma Recurrence." *Medical World News,* July 9, 1984, pp. 9–10.

"Officer Outspoken on Contraception." *American Medical News,* May 25, 1984, pp. 1–31.

O'Reilly, D. "At the Heart of the Matter." *Philadelphia Inquirer,* February 28, 1985, pp. E1, E3.

"Penetration Enhancer Aids Antiherpes Drugs' Actions." *Medical World News,* May 14, 1984, p. 48.

Pepine, C. J., R. L. Feldman, and C. R. Conti. "Action of Intracoronary Nitroglycerin in Refractory Coronary Artery Spasm." *Circulation,* 1982, vol. 65, pp. 411–14.

Polman, D. "The Pill: Debate Over It Took Wing 25 Years Ago." *Philadelphia Inquirer,* May 23, 1985, pp. D1, D8.

"Postponing Preterm Labor with Beta-Adrenergics Can Be Big Cost Saver." *Medical World News,* May 4, 1984, p. 28.

"Pregnancy Vaccine Enters Human Trials." *Medical World News,* January 27, 1986, p. 96.

"Questions Remain About Cyclosporine Link to Posttransplant Malignancies." *Medical World News,* January 9, 1984, pp. 47–48.

Raebel, M. A., J. Black. "The Caffeine Controversy: What Are the Facts?" *Hospital Pharmacy,* 1984, vol. 19, pp. 257–67.

Rensberger, B. "Cancer: The New Synthesis." *Science '84,* September 1984, pp. 28–39.

Robinson, D. H. *The Mircle Finders.* New York: David McKay Co., 1976.

Rosenblatt, S., R. Dodson. *Beyond Valium: The Brave New World of Psychochemistry.* New York: Putnam: 1981.

Schmeck, H. M., Jr. "Cancer-Killing Substance Moves Toward Human Tests." *The New York Times,* June 4, 1985, pp. C1, C5.

"Scientists Say Monoclonal Antibodies May Improve Bladder Cancer Detection." *Medical World News,* June 11, 1984, p. 100.

Shapiro, M., R. P. Charrow. "Scientific Misconduct in Investigational Drug Trials." *New England Journal of Medicine,* 1985, vol. 312, p. 731.

Sherry, S., W. R. Bell, F. H. Duckert, *et al.* "Thrombolytic Therapy in Thrombosis: A National Institutes of Health Consensus Development Conference." *Annals of Internal Medicine,* 1980, vol. 93, pp. 141–44.

Sherry, S. "Personal Reflections on the Development of Thrombolytic Therapy and Its Application to Acute Coronary Thrombosis." *American Heart Journal,* 1981, 102(6–2):1134–39.

Silverman, M., P. R. Lee. *Pill, Profits, & Politics.* Berkeley: University of California Press, 1974.

"Smallpox Is Gone, but Vaccination Lingers On." *Medical World News,* March 2, 1981, p. 19.

Starr, P. *The Social Transformation of American Medicine.* New York: Basic Books, 1982.

Sternbach, H. A., W. Annitto, A. L. C. Pottash, and M. S. Gold. "Anorexic Effects of Naltrexone in Man." *Lancet,* 1982, vol. i, pp. 388–89.

"Sugar and Caffeine Challenges Fail to Support Popular Food-Behavior Link." *Medical World News,* June 11, 1984, p. 107.

Taraxi, R. C. "The Heart in Hypertension." *New England Journal of Medicine,* 1985, vol. 312, pp. 308–09.

"Thalidomide Found to Ease Transplants." *The New York Times,* March 25, 1985, p. C3.

"The Bubble Boy Legacy." *Medical World News,* May 27, 1985, p. 9.

"The Last Word." *AORN Journal,* 1984, vol. 40, p. 302.

"The New Era of Transplants." *Newsweek,* August 29, 1983, p. 38.

"The New Origins of Life." *Time,* September 10, 1984, pp. 46–52.

The Physician's Desk Reference. Oradell, N.J.: Medical Economics Publishing Co., 1985.

"The Pill Takes a Bow on Its 25th." *Medical World News,* January 28, 1985, p. 23.

Thomas, L. *The Youngest Science: Notes of a Medicine-Watcher.* New York: Viking, 1983.

"Tissue-Type Plasminogen Activator Lyses Coronary Thrombi in Minutes." *Medical World News,* January 23, 1984, pp. 17–18.

Toufexis, A., A. Constable, and D. Thompson. "Taming the No. 1 Killer." *Time,* June 1, 1981, pp. 52–58.

Trainor, D. "Canadian Psychiatric Association Brings Together Pioneers in Psychopharmacology." *Psychiatric News,* January 3, 1986, pp. 10–11, 15.

"Tumor-Specific Vaccine Slows Lung Cancer." *Medical World News,* October 28, 1985, p. 66.

"Twenty Discoveries That Changed Our Lives." *Science,* November 1984, pp. 9–190.

"Unstable Angina Patients Continue to Benefit from 12-Week Aspirin Regimen." *Medical World News,* October 22, 1984, p. 25.

Vandam, L. D., J. A. Abbott. "Edward Gilbert Abbott: Enigmatic Figure of the Ether Demonstration." *New England Journal of Medicine,* 1984, vol. 311, pp. 991–94.

Verebey, K., M. S. Gold. "Endorphins and Mental Disease." In: Lajtha, A., ed. *Handbook of Neurochemistry,* vol. 10. New York: Plenum Publishing, 1985.

Walker, K. *The Story of Medicine.* New York: Oxford University Press, 1955.

White, D. J. G., ed. *Cyclosporin A.* New York: Elsevier, 1982.

Williams, H. *Requiem for a Great Killer.* London: Health Horizon, 1973.

Willis, J. "How the Measles Virus Was Done In." *FDA Consumer,* July–August 1982, pp. 11–17.

Ziporyn, T. "Antiepileptics: Age-Old Search for Effective Therapy Continues." *JAMA,* 1985, vol. 254, pp. 329–33.

———. "The Food and Drug Administration: How Those Regulations Came to Be." *JAMA,* 1985, vol. 254, pp. 2037–46.

Zoler, M. L. "Biopharmaceuticals: New Technology Unlocks the Body's Medicine Cabinet." *Medical World News,* March 25, 1985, pp. 40–56.

Index

INDEX

ABOUT THE AUTHOR

Mark S. Gold, M.D., is a psychopharmacologist, psychiatrist, and medical researcher. Dr. Gold and his colleagues at Yale University School of Medicine and Fair Oaks Hospital, Summit, New Jersey, and Boca/Delray, Florida, have made numerous contributions to our understanding of the uses and limitations of wonder drugs. Dr. Gold has authored or co-authored more than 450 papers mainly dealing with three areas of research interest: development of new medical treatments, the role of the laboratory in medicine, and the chemistry of depression. Dr. Gold received his B.A. degree in psychology in 1971 from Washington University, St. Louis, Missouri, and his doctor of medicine in 1975 from the University of Florida College of Medicine, Gainesville. Dr. Gold was a neurobehavioral fellow, resident, chief resident, and faculty member in the Department of Psychiatry at the Yale University School of Medicine.

A Phi Beta Kappa, Dr. Gold was awarded the American Psychiatric Association Foundation's Fund Prize for the discovery of clonidine, the first effective nonaddicting treatment for opiate addicts (1981–1982). He also received the 1982–1983 Presidential Award from the National Association of Private Psychiatric Hospitals for his pioneering research. More recently, he has received (1984–1985) the National Public Service award, Silver Anvil Award, and the National Federation of Parents For a Drug Free Youth award for his cocaine research.

Dr. Gold and co-workers have been pioneers in exploring wonder drugs and have been awarded invention patents for two wonder drugs.

Dr. Gold teaches and lectures at universities and medical societies throughout the United States, and in addition to his research, teaching, and clinical practice, he maintains an active schedule of public service lectures to high school students and parent groups. Dr. Gold has been a guest discussing his research on the "Today Show," "Good Morning America," "CBS Morning News," "The Phil Donahue Show," and many other television shows. Dr. Gold and his work have been the subject of ABC, NBC, CBS, and CNN network news coverage. He has also been the subject of NBC, ABC, Capital Cities Communications, HBO, and CBS specials, and articles by the United Press International, Associated Press, *Time* magazine, *Newsweek*, *Playboy*, and *The New York Times*.